A COUPLE'S GUIDE TO MENOPAUSE

A COUPLE'S GUIDE TO MENOPAUSE

Navigating the Change Together

Kate Usher &
Neil Usher

HERO, AN IMPRINT OF LEGEND TIMES GROUP LTD
51 Gower Street
London WC1E 6HJ
United Kingdom
www.hero-press.com

First published by Hero in 2024

Printed by Akcent Media, 5 The Quay, St Ives, Cambs, PE27 5AR

ISBN (PRINT): 978-1-91505-403-6
ISBN (EBOOK): 978-1-91505-404-3

CONTENTS

TO OUR AMAZING GIRLS

INTRODUCTION

Our relationship began in 2006. We were working for the same organisation and met in the office. We talked a lot, wrote to one another a lot, and when we got together it all progressed very quickly and we were married in 2007. It's been a love affair from the first moment.

We'd been married for three years, together for four, when Kate's menopause began. It's covered almost two thirds of our time together. While it's still in play, lurking in the background, it's been quietened for the time being by hormone replacement therapy (HRT).

That's not to say that during Kate's menopause we didn't experience dark times. Frozen silence, full-bore screamed obscenities (both ways), hateful barbs and seething in opposite corners of the house trying to gather ourselves. It wasn't easy. We made more mistakes along the way than we can possibly recall. Without question, we struggled. But as we were confronted by new symptoms and their impact on the many Kate was already experiencing, we became more able to recognise them for what they were – unwelcome, extremely challenging and at times traumatic. But, importantly, we didn't let the symptoms become our relationship.

If that wasn't enough, it could be imagined that writing a book together may test the tightest bond. But we've talked and shared our way through it as we have with most challenges we've faced or, as in this case, volunteered for.

Kate is now a menopause coach. She founded and runs a successful business advising women and organisations in the corporate world on managing their relationships through the experience, and how organisations can support and retain some of their most brilliant employees. She therefore understands a lot about it. Neil's a regular guy who had to learn quickly and respond to Kate's menopause purposefully. He advises on the design of workplaces and leads complex change projects. It could probably be said that the menopause is a complex change project.

While the menopause has begun to receive coverage in mainstream media, it's still, generally, taboo. Even between couples. Even in progressive circles, where we still don't *like* to talk about it very much. When it's mentioned, it can often provoke a reaction. Therefore, as a society, we elect not to learn much about it. But it remains a privilege to have the option of denial. In many parts of the world, discussing the menopause can be difficult. So, women hide it.

We've seen some menopause coaches and advisers 'invite their partner in' to describe how they provided support and reassurance. Yet these interventions, and so many books on the menopause, still treat it as though something is *wrong*. That it's something to get through, any which way. Yet women can't approach such a significant portion of their lives as *just getting through it*. In taking this approach, it dismisses the potential for all sorts of excitement and adventure that could occur along the way.

Hence the motivation for this book: to share our experience in the hope it'll help others. We don't shy away from the issues, and we tell it as it was and is. We're fully aware that we have the freedom afforded as a couple to be as open as possible about the menopause, and we're going to make the most of it.

While it's true that two to six per cent of men in their late 40s to early 50s experience the andropause, resulting in a range of symptoms brought on by an abnormal decline in testosterone level that's relatively easily medicated, 100 per cent of women have a menopause, and it represents a significant biological change. Their partner is going to be involved whether they like it or not.

And so, this is a book about managing the menopause together, written by us both. While this book is based on our experience in a heterosexual relationship, there will be elements that are applicable irrespective of gender identity or sexual orientation.

The book takes eight aspects of the menopause and looks at each from the female and male perspective. There are similarities and differences. It offers insight and suggestions as to what we might do based on over a decade of direct personal experience of the menopause. It's three books in one: the female view, the male view, and the joint view. We've kept it grounded and real, and had a bit of fun with it too.

We're not medical doctors nor clinically trained in any regard. There's no medical advice contained in this book. If this is what you're seeking, depending on where you live, we recommend you consult your doctor. They may in turn refer you to a specialist menopause clinic.

We're not offering an academic textbook. Yet we're aware that data and evidence sources are important. At the end of the book, you'll find details about where key facts and assertions have been obtained, together with suggested further reading if you wish to explore some of the issues raised in more depth.

We recognise that the unique nature of the experience for every woman will mean that some of what we offer will be helpful and work, while some won't. Similarly, there may be other approaches that have – or will – work for you that we haven't covered. We're all still learning.

We hope you enjoy reading this book and get something out of it. Preferably together.

Kate Usher & Neil Usher
January 2024

A COUPLE'S GUIDE TO MENOPAUSE

1

WHAT IS THE MENOPAUSE?

An understanding of what the menopause is, how long it lasts and how it changes over time is vital grounding for the rest of this book.

Before we share our experiences and advice, a basic understanding of the menopause will be useful – one that looks at the symptoms and addresses the essential issues. To make it easy to follow, we've set it out as a Q&A (questions and answers). This is all public-domain information, but as with many matters we'll discuss, it's not so much that it's 'out there'; it's just that it's not often organised in a way that makes it easy for us to find, access and validate. We'll refer again to this chapter as we go, so it may be worth dropping a sticky note in.

WHO GETS A MENOPAUSE?

Every female, transgender man and some non-binary people will have a menopause. It comes with having ovaries. It's a biological fact.

WHY DOES THE MENOPAUSE HAPPEN?

The menopause sits between the two phases of womanhood. While there are various complex endocrinological suggestions, due to a woeful lack of research, there is little understanding of what exactly causes a woman's menopause to begin. What we do know is that once it does, a woman's steady cyclical production of oestrogen, progesterone and testosterone (yes, women have that too; in fact at times, they have more than men) goes haywire, which brings about the symptoms.

WHAT HAPPENS DURING THE MENOPAUSE?

There are three phases to the menopause: the warm-up act (perimenopause), followed by the main event (the menopause itself), and the warm-down (post-menopause). It begins, happens, and peters out. It's here we start to get used to the uncertainty and unpredictability of the whole experience.

Perimenopause is when symptoms start to show themselves.

There's no rule as to how long it lasts, but current thinking suggests around four years. If a woman is still fertile at this stage and therefore she may still get pregnant. If you're trying to get pregnant at this stage, don't lose hope; if you're trying not to, continue to take precautions.

The menopause itself lasts a calendar year. It's when a woman hasn't had a period for a full twelve months. Which means determining that it's happened is only possible afterwards (especially as, for most women, this is a time of unpredictable periods).

If a woman gets to eleven and a half months and has a period, it wasn't the menopause, and the guessing begins all over again.

When the year has passed, the woman then becomes 'postmenopausal'. Symptoms may continue for some time postmenopause. Again, this has no fixed term.

WHEN DOES THE MENOPAUSE HAPPEN?

Menopause symptoms usually occur between the ages of 45 and 55. The average age of the *actual* menopause (twelve months since a woman's last period) is between 49 and 51 depending on ethnicity. If 45 seems surprisingly young, it is. Remember that thought.

It's important to state that 5 per cent of women have their menopause before the age of 45, and 1 per cent before 40. Although rare, it includes very young women in their teens and their 20s. 'Medical menopause' happens when the menopause is brought on by a medical treatment and can occur at any age.

HOW LONG DOES THE MENOPAUSE LAST?

There are many views on how long the whole menopause lasts, given that it's an entirely personal experience. It's usually estimated at between four and eight years of symptoms over all three phases. Yet it remains unpredictable and variable, complicated by the potential for symptoms to fade in and out. It can sometimes take years for women to piece together their symptoms and to be able to confirm it's happening.

At eight years that's around a tenth of an average lifespan, over a fifth of a career. Some people worry that a common cold lasts a fortnight and feels like forever.

WHAT ARE THE SIGNS IT'S ARRIVED?

Here's where the fun really starts. Different fun, naturally. There's a myth that everything kicks off with an all-fires-blazing hot flush. While this is true for some, for a significant number it's not. In many ways it's easier for those who experience hot flushes because they're immediately recognisable, being an unusual occurrence in everyday pre-menopausal life.

Commonly, women start to recognise that something simply *isn't right*. This may reveal itself through anxiety, moods, shorter temper or forgetfulness, for example. Self-awareness and a knowledge of the symptoms listed are the essential keys to diagnosis.

WHAT ARE THE SYMPTOMS?

The symptoms are, at a rudimentary level, both physical and psychological. Here's the list. There are over 40 of them:

PHYSICAL

Allergies	Insomnia
Breast pain	Irregular periods
Brittle nails	Itchy skin (formication)
Changes in body odour	Joint pain
Cold flushes	Loss of muscle mass
Digestive problems	Migraines
Dizziness	Night sweats
Dry hair	Dry eyes
Dry skin	Recurrent UTIs
Fatigue	Sleep apnoea
Flooding	Snoring
Gum problems	Stiff joints
Hair loss	Tinnitus
Hot flushes	Unwanted hair growth
Incontinence (stress and urge)	Weight gain
Increased thrush	Vaginal atrophy/dryness

PSYCHOLOGICAL

Anxiety	Loss of verbal recall
Depression	Memory lapses
Difficulty concentrating	Mood swings
Loss of confidence	Panic attacks
Loss of sex drive	

As items on a list, they give no hint of relative impact or scale. Anxiety can have devastating, wide-ranging and life-changing effects. Snoring, however, is just annoying for anyone in earshot; unless it's keeping a partner awake who has a critical job and whose performance begins to suffer with negative consequences for those with whom they're in contact – tricky when they're a brain surgeon or fly a space shuttle.

Certain symptoms are triggers for others. They're not neatly packaged units. Night sweats contribute to a lack of sleep, which in turn causes, or makes worse, mood swings and loss of concentration. Similarly, depression and loss of confidence may result in tiredness and loss of libido. In turn, loss of libido may cause or worsen depression. The relationship between symptoms is complex and always changing.

DO ALL WOMEN EXPERIENCE THE SAME MENOPAUSE?

The menopause for every woman is as unique as her fingerprint. Unpredictability comes as standard.

WHAT IS THE MENOPAUSE?

As a basic guide: a quarter of women will have virtually no awareness of their menopause other than variable periods. Half of women will have some symptoms that, with a few lifestyle changes and support, they'll be able to manage, with a little inconvenience. The remaining quarter will have a traumatic and life-changing experience and will require considerable support. Women can't predict or choose which group they belong to.

HOW DO THE SYMPTOMS CHANGE?

They can and they do change, in terms of the range, severity and duration of each – one by one or all at the same time. Which makes anticipating what comes next, and how to plan to deal with them, incredibly hard. It does depend on how they're managed, as those at the 'core' can influence the severity or impact of others. But some symptoms seem to remain constant throughout unless specific support is obtained. They include hot flushes and night sweats, insomnia, anxiety and depression.

HOW TO GET HELP?

There are four areas. First, asking others and sharing in return can be helpful and reassuring. It makes the menopause feel normal and helps remove the mystery, stigma and, importantly, the isolation that's often felt.

Second, there's a lot of great advice and guidance online, but as with everything online it does need investigation. Talking and sharing can help with what's found, too. Kate's YouTube channel (Kate Usher Menopause Coach) is a great place to start.

Third, for specific issues or approaches, qualified and registered specialists should always be used. Whether they be nutritionists, herbalists, naturopaths, counsellors, coaches, psychotherapists or gynaecologists, it'll make a difference if they have a proven specialism in menopause.

Lastly, the health service in your country of residence. Doctors' practices often have a women's health specialist. A referral to a local menopause clinic is a possibility. Many countries have an official society from whom support or recommendations can be obtained. The British Menopause Society and the North American Menopause Society are examples, whose websites contain lists of state and private specialists by area.

HOW DOES IT END?

The menopause doesn't end as such; it fades. Like the way it begins, it relies on an awareness of things starting to settle down and symptoms easing. Where once there was a feeling that things weren't quite right, the sensation of balance begins to return. There are some symptoms that can continue for some time after the rest have departed. They include, but are not limited to, hot flushes, anxiety, sleep problems and vaginal dryness.

IS THERE ANY GOOD NEWS?

Yes. Kate had an awful menopause, but while not without significant challenges, we still lived a full life throughout and did many of the things we used to do before it arrived – essentially because we were adamant that we would carry on, whatever it threw at us.

Whether it's you who's menopausal or you're the male partner of a menopausal woman, you need to know that it's manageable; that life will continue for the duration, and that when it's over there's an incredible second phase to live and enjoy. That's a lot of good news.

2

PERCEPTIONS

The outdated and prejudicial way in which the menopause is portrayed in society skews our perception of what it is, how we might manage it and what comes afterwards.

PERCEPTIONS: KATE

TWO TALES AND AN ADDENDUM

There are two stories and an addendum generally told about the menopause.

First, that it's a living hell. That it'll ravage us, and as women we have no choice but to put up with it, after which we can withdraw to a sedate and unchallenging meander to the end of our life, sexless and quite possibly alone.

Or, that it's nothing to be concerned about at all. That our mothers and grandmothers navigated it without any fuss, and that we should button up and deal with whatever it throws at us. After which we can withdraw to a sedate and unchallenging meander to the end of our life, sexless and quite possibly alone.

Added to this is the unspoken belief that men aren't involved, that it's for women to deal with. Alone.

Neither story nor the addendum is right.

THE REALITY

The story that *should* be told is that the menopause is a hugely variable experience for all women, about which we're learning all the time, and that if you have a partner – we'll assume for the purpose of this book that you do – they have a key role in helping us manage the journey, after which, we'll enjoy a vibrant, energised, sexual future in which we're in full control of our choices and decisions. With our partner. Should we wish it.

DECEPTION AND COERCION

As the real story is very different from those repeatedly told, we need to address our perceptions of the menopause and of menopausal women. We must actively counter the big, scary monster of a lie in all areas of society that menopause is an old white woman's condition, the gateway to retirement, invisibility and celibacy.

If we search online for *menopausal women*, the images we're supplied are all too often white women in their 60s and 70s, looking broken. They're portrayed as frumpy, difficult, sweaty, desperate and a little mad, somehow obsolete and therefore invisible. Depictions of menopausal women during our 40s and 50s, the typical menopausal years, are absent. It's unsurprising, therefore, that we fear the menopause. A woman said to me recently: "I want a supermodel to represent me, not them."

THE FALLOUT

I've had people say to me "it's just a picture/advert/TV programme/film – it's not real. Don't you think you're being overdramatic?"

But by visually excluding swathes of society – that is, anyone who's not white and in their 60s – we're excluding them from the pathway to support. Which is categorically wrong.

Because the images we're given depict considerably older women than those who are entering perimenopause, it can take years for some women to recognise the symptoms for what they are, believing they're too young. Over those years relationships, careers and self-esteem can be utterly devastated. It's a similar situation for women from minority groups, who can feel excluded from many channels of support.

Very young women in their teens and twenties who have premature ovarian insufficiency (POI) suffer prejudice and ridicule at every turn. As much as it's difficult to see a woman 20 years older than us representing us, imagine how it feels for that person to be over 40 years older?

When it comes to revealing we're menopausal to our partner, and to our family, friends or colleagues for that matter, many of us fear that those images will dance across their minds and change people's perception of us as we utter the word 'menopause'. That we'll age, become difficult, be less able and, in the case of our partner, less attractive. We fear it because these images are so ingrained in our societal perception that we have had to tussle with them, too. For some it's fleeting, for others it's a roadblock.

Lastly, the consistent use of older women to depict menopause can reinforce the negative stereotype in some men's minds, to a degree sufficient to trigger a need to exit their relationship for a younger, unsuspecting candidate. The perception can also ensure that such behaviour is considered acceptable and understandable by those around them.

HISTORY REPEATS ITSELF

There's a very simple reason for this lazy thinking. Women born around the turn of the last century were the first generation to experience menopause as standard rather than the exception. But only just. With a life expectancy of 52, it was an end-of-life experience. Life was extremely hard for most, with poor living standards and nutrition, numerous pregnancies, the difficult challenge of rearing children without modern gadgets (notably, the automatic washing machine) and common diseases we don't even think about now. By the time they reached their late 40s to early 50s these women looked like women do today in their 60s and 70s.

I have a photograph of my paternal grandmother when she was 51. She looked about 70 and died within a year of it being taken. Seven children, six surviving, brought up in a Glaswegian tenement (small flat), a husband with a long-term illness, fighting to make ends meet, all three sons conscripted, one killed in service. Is there any wonder that the years took their toll?

As much as our knowledge of menopause is limited today, these women would have known very little other than rumour and whisper.

Physically they'd have suffered. From multiple pregnancies, women's vaginas would have been torn to shreds and prolapses must have been extremely common. Not for them Kegel exercises or gentle stitching to ensure the beauty and function of their femininity. Vaginal dryness would have either been endured or ended intimacy for a lack of understanding. Couples would have struggled to start the conversation or find products to help. Flooding, constant urinary tract infections (UTIs), thrush and incontinence would have made life extremely difficult and intimacy embarrassing. If we find conversations about these matters awkward today, imagine them back then.

The psychological symptoms that we're only just starting to discuss would have been cloaked in the negative Victorian view of mental ill-health. Women who suffered from depression, anxiety, panic attacks, mood swings, rage and memory loss would likely have feared the Gothic towers of mental institutions.

It was bleak.

It's not surprising our grandmothers taught our mothers, and ultimately us, to fear menopause, to talk in only the darkest of corners. In fact, most of us grew up only knowing it as the monster that is 'The Change'.

Men weren't included in the development of even this rudimentary level of awareness. It was considered nothing to do with them, by women and men alike.

All these elements have created the legacy we're battling with today. We're still applying the experience, awareness and thinking of our grandmothers' generation to the conversation, and how we're visually depicted.

BREAKING THE MOULD

But the present generation of menopausal women is unusual in that we're a cohort of firsts. Of course, there were a few preceding exceptions, naturally – but as a generation we've broken the mould. We're the first to get an education, a career and financial independence as standard. We're the first to have children while holding down a career, and now to have our menopause while working as well. As a generation we've pushed through barriers, developed higher expectations and demanded a different way of being. We're prepared to stand up for what we know to be right, and for our rights.

While there's much still wrong with the world of work for women, from inequality to physical and emotional threat, we can state with confidence that as a generation we're the menopause upstarts. And we're only just beginning.

GUILTY AS CHARGED

If only it were that easy.

As women we judge ourselves and each other extremely harshly. How we dress, behave and carry ourselves comes under continual scrutiny. Our reproductive characteristics fare no different. If we've had an easy time with our periods, we negatively view those who don't. We judge one another on how we manage fertility, pregnancy, childbirth – natural, medical or C-section – and then how we raise our children. As women, we'll all at some point have been both critical and criticised. We all know it's true.

When a woman judges another woman in this way, we're reinforcing the negative stereotype and supercharging the tales that we've been told.

It feels like the greatest betrayal of all, that we can't even rely on other women to show us empathy. If we're ever going to change this narrative, we need to stop demeaning each other and amplify a new perspective. There are several ways we can do this.

🎬 KATE'S ACTION PLAN

EXERCISE OUR POWER

We must recognise our power as consumers. When we've seen how we're misrepresented, we can't unsee it. Women today in their 40s and 50s are vibrant, brilliant, driven and formidable. We're the first generation to have disposable income at this age and, yes, we want to spend it – but not on 24-hour girdles, Crimplene and cleaning products. We have power in our liquidity. It's time to demand of those brands that sell to us that we're represented accurately. It's time to turn our backs on them. Demand more: money talks.

WHY?

- We're talking about skincare products that use models in their 70s for menopause-specific products. Or fashion brands that use teenage girls to model clothes aimed at women over 40. It's demeaning and offensive.
- The other market that is growing rapidly is menopause fashion. This is predominantly focused on cooling fabrics for hot flushes. Most women I know aged in their 40s and 50s still want to look fabulous. They haven't given up. Yet many of these products reinforce a dowdy view of women that should be long gone.
- The menopause market is predicted to reach $24.4 billion globally. We have more influence than we seem

to think. We can drive the narrative through choice and vocalisation.

SUPPORT, DON'T JUDGE

We have to get over ourselves. It's time we stopped colluding with the tales too often told, and recognise that every woman's experience is different. Women need support at this time, not judgement.

WHY?

- We're all doing the best we can, with the resources we have available. Judgement isn't helpful, especially when it comes from another woman.
- Bias is part of the human condition, conscious as much as unconscious. We all have and display it. As uncomfortable as this admission may be, unless we face it, we block the opportunity to change the way we think or behave.
- If we're lucky enough to be one of the quarter of women who sail through their menopause without any issues, we must be grateful while recognising that it's not the case for other women. If a woman must take HRT because her life is literally falling apart, we can't assume it's because they haven't got a grip of themself or made the lifestyle changes we believe they needed to.

TELL THE RIGHT STORY

We need to know, tell and retell the *right* story about meno-pause. Given the journey to this point, it's unhelpful that the media are still representing us in a way that's outmoded and – let's face it – derogatory. They're applying age-based imagery to us that was applicable nearly a century ago. It needs to be called out. It's important to note that it's per-petuated not just by men, but by women too.

WHY?

- These images and portrayals make us question ourselves and wonder whether we're actually less than we are; that time's up, and that our usefulness is defined by the effectiveness of our ovaries rather than the incredible wealth of knowledge and ability that we carry within us.
- If we don't openly and proactively reject the myths we hear, read and see every day, they will persist. It's in our hands.
- I'm yet to meet a woman where I'm not in awe of her strength and ability to face adversity, no matter her background and circumstances. Division merely perpetuates the status quo. Changing the way the world perceives us requires a togetherness, a unity of purpose. It's entirely possible.

INCLUDE MEN

We must ensure that we include men in our conversations, whether that be our partner, children, family, friends or colleagues. They're not separate, neither are they excluded from the impact of our symptoms. If we're to bring men along with us in this area of life, we have to ensure they're part of the solution and talk about it.

WHY?

- Educating men in what menopause is, in its many forms, means we're creating the opportunity for them to support us in every context.
- Our partners want to support us and will step forward when they understand. This makes them better friends, fathers and colleagues too. As they talk about it, other men will be educated and in turn step forward. We'll create momentum.
- The opportunity for incremental change is considerable when it includes men's contribution. We need to capitalise on it.

o o o

How we perceive menopause has a wide-reaching impact on us as women, our relationships, our career and our long-term wellbeing. It has a societal impact, too. While it might feel like too big an issue to transform, we can all contribute to the change that's needed. We just need to start. Today.

PERCEPTIONS: NEIL

ALL THAT WE SEE

Menopause is what it is, and what we see. It may even be, as some have claimed, that menopause – as with everything in life – is *only* what we see, and that there isn't any other reality at all. Which is why consideration of the way we see menopause is located right at the start of this book.

You've probably gathered from Kate's views that if we could fix one thing that would improve the prospects of menopausal women, it would be the recognition and reversal of the negative way it's perceived. By almost everyone.

This may be a surprising claim, given the focus on managing symptoms that characterises much of the present coverage of menopause. If you've reached the start of your partner's menopause fully loaded with fear and negativity, it's understandable. At the start of Kate's menopause, we both had too.

AND SO IT GOES AROUND

The story of the menopause is buried in a bigger story of men and women. It's a ridiculous, dangerous and damaging story. It's not my story, far from it, but it's what we're fed. Sometimes subtly, sometimes quite literally. It runs like this:

In this story, women are shown as having a very clear life cycle based around their ability to reproduce. This has two aspects – desirability as a mate, and the ability to bear healthy children. Women are depicted as reaching a physical peak in both respects from their 20s to mid-30s. It all slowly begins to slip (or sag) from there through to their 50s. By which time, if they're still holding their own among the younger generations in peak fertility, it's the result of infills, surgery, a safe life, incredibly good fortune or literally a fortune. After that, it's rather irrelevant. All of which perpetuates misogyny as a regrettable feature of modern society.

Also in this story, men keep on winning. In their 20s they're full of youthful vigour, strength, determination; they're a coiled spring, making up for their lack of worldly experience with pure, pent-up cheeky potential. Yet as they age, striding effortlessly through the decades, accumulating wealth, partners, overseas properties and soft-top sports cars, hair greying at the temples, laughter lines and scars telling a thousand tales, they're still fertile, viable, and downright unbelievably and irresistibly sexy. 'Silver foxes' being the generic term used: 'silver' for their hair, 'fox' for their nocturnal cunning and tendency to leave a mess behind them for others to clear up.

These views are repugnant, but everywhere. Nested within this story like a Matryoshka doll lies the story of the menopause. Thereafter we're offered us a portrayal of women as grey (not silver) and diminished, destined to see out the remainder of their days in gentle pursuits.

However absurd that whole depiction seems, it's all too often how mass media and the arts reinforce the perception of menopausal women even when they're attempting to suggest it's not the case. Showing an actual 45-year-old woman simply doesn't fit the popular narrative of menopausal women being *past it*. It's ingrained, born not just of an outdated view of the menopause, but even more importantly, a void of understanding of what comes afterwards. The second phase of womanhood.

We can throw up our arms and claim: "It's not like that!" No, it may actually be worse than that. I'm erring on the side of caution here.

I PERCEIVE, THEREFORE I AM

Perceptions create mental models that drive behaviour. As the menopause arrives unannounced in their partner's life, and hence their own, men have the ultimate cop-out available to them: *to walk away*. To simply opt for a younger woman, one not yet facing or struggling with the menopause. And they can continue to do so for as long as possible to never have to face it – just simply keep trading younger. Because as an 'older man', society still acknowledges that it's perfectly acceptable to seek women more junior.

The other way around, of course – the younger man, older woman scenario – is part of the same master story but perceived as going against the natural order of things, in which the woman is irresponsible at best, verging on being in desperate denial of the twilight of her desirability. A man having children with multiple partners over several decades is considered a rogue, a woman doing so is – well – we can all fill in the rest. Our views of boys and girls in their earliest years – boys experimenting, causing havoc and getting away with it; girls being polite, impeccably behaved, responsible and dignified – plays out throughout our lifetime.

Much of men's perception of the menopause is often non-existent. Unless directly affected by our partner's menopause or that of a family member, friend or work colleague, there will have been no compelling reason to understand it. Or even to acknowledge it's a thing. It only made it on to the curriculum in England in 2020.

Of course, we as men may believe the more convenient of the two stories of the menopause that Kate described: that because women knuckle down and just get on with it, rarely talking about it for fear of owning up to the end of their biological (and by implication societal) usefulness, it can't be that bad a deal, justifying male disinterest. And so, the myth goes around.

There appears to be no logic as to why this negative perception of the menopause has taken hold, other than fear: either of the actuality, or the unknown. Or potentially for men that an army of fearsome and fearless post-menopausal women would upset the comfortably patriarchal way of things.

What men might do regarding perceptions has to be seen

within the broader context of where the menopause fits in to our entire view of the male and female life cycle. Most things in life are stacked in men's favour, within systems designed to keep them that way. It's easy therefore to let them remain so, even if giving the appearance of demanding the balance be redressed: a bit of social media outrage now and then, a little positive discrimination at work, perhaps. While there should be many other contexts for men to open their minds to the menopause, nothing focusses the mind on the need for change quite like having daughters and considering their education and opportunities.

🎬 NEIL'S ACTION PLAN

KNOW OUR STUFF

Men need to educate themselves. Even with the basics: being aware of what the menopause is, how it affects women and the age at which it occurs. We can take it as far as we wish from this point: no one's expecting us to get a PhD in post-reproductive health studies. But we must defy the view that knowing about the menopause is for women only. It's for everyone.

WHY?

- We can't begin to see and respond to the challenge of stereotyped gender stories until we at least know the facts. And they are *facts*, not opinions.

- It'll give us the confidence to challenge. A challenger mindset is a critical feature of a menopausal partner. We'll encounter damaging and negative myths and stereotypes everywhere, during and afterwards, and will need to be able to refute them in an informed way.

REWRITE THE NEGATIVE STUFF

We have a part to play in rewriting the story as it should be through positive intervention. In not accepting what we're fed. How? By recognising the problem (however uncomfortable this may be), actively calling it out at every opportunity and even simply speaking about it. Not just the menopausal aspects, the broader story in which the menopause exists. The menopause is a fantastic place to start.

WHY?

- It's a judgement we must make, in terms of what's important and how we handle collective prejudice. It may create some awkward moments in the company of male friends and colleagues, even to the extent of jeopardising those relationships. But if it does, are they the relationships we want?
- It's not a suggestion that every sexist comment uttered in our midst be taken outside, but the rollback must start somewhere. And as Kate stated, where it's a societal problem, *we are society*.

TAKE IT TO THE SECOND PHASE

The combination of awareness and positive intervention must extend to the second phase of women's lives, beyond menopause. Men are predominantly unaware of what happens for women when the menopause is over beyond the popular portrayal of a gentle withdrawal.

WHY?

- We'll need to challenge these perceptions, too, that for women it's all done bar the jam-making (with apologies if you make excellent jam). As we'll find as we explore the material available about the menopause, it's almost entirely about *getting through it*. We cover what the second phase is and means at the end of this book. Not just for completeness – it's essential.
- We'll need to be ready for when it happens. The point is made several times through this book that life for our partner won't revert to a 'normal' pre-menopausal state. As we'll cover in the last chapter, they'll be different. And so, too, will we need to be. It's another phase of our lives, and our lives together too.

o o o

If we think we can be a positive influence and contributor at home while we happily prop up and echo existing prejudice and misinformation elsewhere, we're kidding ourselves. Our taking an active role in shifting societal perceptions of the menopause lets our partner know we're on their side and fully prepared to get involved. We must be able to contribute at all levels. We'll reveal ourselves soon enough to our partner if we can't or won't.

As men still have the lion's share of power, control and influence, an incredible opportunity presents itself here. We could actually be the ones to drive this change. Which means we need to reject the idea that in taking the opportunity, it would be an 'own goal'. Imagine the potency of men inviting and encouraging women to talk about the menopause from a position of enlightenment, actively rejecting and campaigning against negative and outdated stereotypes of all genders at all ages. What do we think?

3

TALKING

Talking and listening are vital in any relationship, but are particularly so during the menopause, when a commitment to learn, adapt, share and respond openly together can make a hugely beneficial difference.

TALKING: KATE

Talking is the foundation of every great relationship, whether platonic or romantic, and however deep. We can have all the other stuff – the chemistry, spirituality, common experience, physical attraction, soul connection – but at some point, we're going to have to say something to one another and listen when the other talks.

SELF-TALK

Yes, we all talk to ourselves. It's our inner voice, where talking about the menopause begins. Often, we're not even conscious of it and so don't hear it.

For many women the initial stages of perimenopause are full of dismissal. Our inner voice tells us it's something else, or nothing. In fact, until we get our first hot flush, many women, and doctors for that matter, fail to identify this phase of life. Which, of course, makes it extremely tricky for those women who never get a hot flush.

I can say this with confidence because I spent four years reasoning away the mounting number of psychological and cognitive symptoms I was experiencing. I simply had no awareness of what was happening.

It can be a slow process of joining the dots – mood swings, loss of libido, insomnia and hair that's suddenly turned from lush to straw – before we realise what's driving all the issues. However, we eventually work it out.

WOMAN TO WOMAN

When we talk to other women, if it's about a biological subject, it's fertility: whether we have time, if we consider that it's running out, or whether we want to exercise it at all. We don't seem to marry the end of fertility with the menopause. Or at least don't choose to.

As already mentioned, the menopause has considerable societal baggage. The menopause wasn't openly discussed by our mothers or grandmothers. The sense of embarrassment, even shame, around its onset meant little more than a knowing glance passed from woman to woman, generation to generation.

Added to which, the sense of isolation and loneliness created by menopausal symptoms further lessens the chances of the menopause being discussed between us. We instinctively think it best to talk about something else. Or not at all.

In the past, men weren't even included in the knowing glances. And yet it's our partner we now need to open up to about our menopause.

LIFE GETS IN THE WAY

In our relationship, we often get out of the habit of creating time for talking. Life gets in the way: work, possibly kids, friends, family and all manner of associated other pursuits. After all, who has any spare time? If any emerges, we'll fill it with other activities, things that need doing. Most of us barely have time to shave our armpits.

By talking, I don't mean sorting out logistics and arrangements, but a mutually respectful and interested sharing of ideas, thoughts and needs. I grew up in a household where my parents never talked, not even to argue. Their only conversation revolved around what was for tea, the need to buy more dog food or establishing who needed to take me to or pick me up from swimming twice a day. It was sterile and ended in a bitter divorce. I promised myself this wouldn't happen to me.

This is both Neil's and my second marriage. Obviously, I tripped up on the above promise first time around. Neil admits to the same. This is why talking is one of our great indulgences. We delight in time to talk. Which is lucky because the menopause drives a need to talk, a lot. Not only to reveal what's going on, but also to discuss its impact and how we'll manage it together. Please note, I did say *together*. While it's undoubtedly for each woman *her* own personal menopause, it is, by its very nature, a shared experience.

MIND READER?

Which brings us to the next issue. I find telepathy makes my head hurt. Partners can't read our minds. They're on the outside wondering what on earth has happened to the steady, proportionate, cheerful and philosophical person we used to be. OK, most of the time.

We'll cover some of the more common issues later in this book, but for now we need to focus on the unreasonable female expectation that our partner should simply know and understand what's happening. Because *for heaven's sake* they should. But they don't and won't.

Just like we all do when we don't know what's happening, they'll be making assumptions about what's driving this change in us and (as Neil will also reference) making up a whole heap of nonsense.

SOMETHING TO DECLARE

Some of us at this point will start to feel slightly sick at having to declare that we're menopausal. The most common reason for this is that women fear that the person they hope will love and desire them forever will, in that moment, see them shrivel like a prune before their eyes. Whatever regime of self-care and health we've pursued, we fear that the menopause instantly ages us. Not just in terms of perception, which we just covered, but in real terms. Suddenly they see us as the images in the media portray us. They may even look harder for the evidence to prove the hunch.

If we want to keep our relationship and nurture it so that when we get to the other end of this we're still a loved-up (and, most of us hope, sexed-up) team of two, the only option is to talk about it. And because the menopause goes on for years, we'll need to talk about it again and again. This is not a once-and-done activity.

I found that the conversations I had with Neil were a way for me to gain clarity of what was going on and how we were managing. Or not. They were a confirmation that we were and are still in this together. It became as important for me as it was for him and the unity of our family.

WHEN IT'S NOT THAT EASY

But not everyone has a partner that wants to, or is prepared to, talk. Some of us live in an environment where emotional or intimate conversations are either frowned upon or simply not part of our day-to-day behaviour.

I understand, but the menopause doesn't.

Our symptoms are out there, like children ransacking a sweet shop, getting more extreme as they go. Ultimately, we won't be able to keep them hidden, some or all will slip out. Our partner, no matter how uncommunicative, will be able to see it as well and will want to know what's happening.

For those who simply have not learnt to talk inside relationships, I can say from experience that the drive to be with our partner forces us to start talking.

CONFUSION

Many of us will find that we need to start talking before we understand fully what's going on. We'll know that we're acting differently, maybe unreasonably or have a shorter fuse. We might have gone off sex completely. We might feel concerned about our relationship, or be consumed by fear about the direction in which we ourselves are heading, or possibly even flicking between the two. This, unsurprisingly, raises anxiety and stress (see the chapter on 'Moods') and aggravates our symptoms. But the fact that you're reading this book says that you've at least considered attributing the changes in yourself to the menopause.

Once my physical symptoms started, I knew what they were, and that Neil needed to be as aware as I was. Which at the time was not very aware at all. I think I told him and then had a hot flush in front of him as I was speaking. Although he was surprised and concerned, he quickly understood where we were. He really had little choice, as thereafter the hot flushes came thick and fast. I think I melted over breakfast, lunch, dinner and everything in between. It really was a baptism of fire, for both of us.

We learnt as we went along. I began researching the menopause simply because I had no explanation, no list of symptoms to check against and I needed to know. As each symptom or group of symptoms arrived, I needed the reassurance for myself and then from Neil that this was all part of the same thing. Here's what we can do to get the conversation going.

▶ KATE'S ACTION PLAN

ADMISSION

We have to start with us. We must recognise and admit that our menopause is happening before we do so to others, so that we can take control of our experience. We can map the symptoms we're experiencing using the list in this book. We'll then have much-needed perspective and ultimately a route forward. We can practice talking and listening on ourselves first.

WHY?

- Many women take time to identify this phase of life for what it is. The earlier we do so, the better. It can take some women years. Some will have visited the doctor numerous times and received treatment for individual symptoms which persisted regardless. Others will be caught out by a massive step change, from irritable minor symptoms to traumatic emotional tsunamis. The latter can occur at any point in the transition, even post-menopause.
- We can't talk to our partner about the menopause with any intent until we've had the conversation with ourselves, or it may get messy. We want our partner to support us, not to try and untangle our denials.

TIME AND PLACE

If the thought of talking about our symptoms with our partner is causing dread, it's time to get organised. Once we know what's going on, it's time to think about when and where we're going to start the conversation.

WHY?

- It may seem obvious, but if we feel crap in the mornings, it's best not to try to talk about things in the morning. Similarly, if we're exhausted in the evening and our emotions are frazzled, it's really not the time for a heart-to-heart. We and they don't need the added stress.

- In terms of place, we're best to be somewhere private, where we won't be interrupted or overheard. We'll bring others in if or when we need. No one else needs to see our discomfort in real time while we test the water. This applies to kids as well; we can always speak to them later. If things descend into an argument or finger-pointing, we'll need to stop, walk away and come back to it another time. But not give up.

AWARENESS

Starting the conversation with our partner requires a baseline awareness on both our parts – preferably the same baseline, so we're drawing on a familiar knowledge pool. The opening chapter of this book may be a helpful reference point, particularly the symptoms list. Of course, we'll need to build our awareness first, but we'll need to have the information for our partner with us when we begin.

WHY?

- Having facts available builds instant confidence between us.
- Even if we've investigated the menopause in much more detail by the time we talk, it'll be helpful initially to keep the conversation centred around the facts we present and share, so it feels like common ground.

- It's not unusual for our partner to be aware of a symptom affecting us before we do. Sometimes we're blindsided by what's happening. The information will help identify them.
- This is not a static experience. We'll have to keep returning to the list as we go through our menopause. Things can and do change.

MOMENTUM

Once we start, we must talk about talking. We have to tell our partner what we want to talk about, our path to understanding what's going on and what we're doing about it. Then, we need to provide the opportunity for them to give their reaction and to ask questions.

WHY?

- It's likely to come as a relief to our partner that there's a reason we've changed or are behaving differently.
- Talking will be a prompt for action. We need to have thought about what it is we're going to ask our partner to do and be confident they'll be able to do it quickly, easily and repeatedly. We need to think about the symptoms that impact us in ways where support can be both provided and potentially effective. Some we'll have to deal with ourselves. If we're asking our partner to metaphorically climb mountains and swim oceans to help us, they'll try to do it once, maybe twice, complain, check out, and that's

it. This will be demoralising for us *and* them. We need to make it easy so that both of us will benefit.

EVIDENCE

As our conversations progress, we must show our partner that their support works – the before and after – to close the loop with visible evidence.

WHY?

- If we're saying their support works but they can't see it, they won't consider their efforts are of benefit and may stop.
- We're far more likely to embed open and regular talking in our relationship if it's producing results that we can both recognise. They become a talking point themselves.
- There's no downside to evidence.

o o o

Talking gets easier the more we do it. We need to start somewhere, and starting is often the hardest part. If we understand where we are and what we need, we're able to talk and to strengthen the bond between us. Silence serves no purpose. That and the 'not knowing' are toxic to relationships; in this instance they're completely unnecessary. It's entirely possible to talk our way out of the shadows together.

TALKING: NEIL

Over many years, when it comes to conversation within a relationship, two male traits have been lampooned in popular culture. As with most such depictions, despite being for comic effect, they contain a kernel of truth. Neither help when it comes to supporting a partner through their menopause. If both are evident in a relationship, it might be considered lucky to have survived. Or, perhaps, unlucky. Strangely, they're almost opposites: not talking, and talking rubbish.

SOUNDS OF SILENCE

The first trait concerns men's apparent active avoidance within relationships of both talking and listening. A great deal of this may have a basis in our upbringing. We may recognise some of the following:

- We've watched our own fathers and grandfathers, when anything tricky arises, master the art of avoidance, and been taught that, as men, it's what we do.
- We've been bullied, or seen our friends bullied, at school and through early manhood for not only talking about feelings but *actually daring to have any feelings in the first place*. Feelings mean vulnerability, even failure – traits that aren't 'manly'.

- We've been exposed to influences that portray the 'hero' as the strong, ultimately moral (often after several dubious decisions) but silent type.
- When under any form of pressure, we've been repeatedly told to 'man up', a primitive form of resilience we may today recognise as bloodless self-harm.

But somehow, even though we've slowly become more open to the idea of difficult conversations, we always seem to be a huge stride behind women in this regard.

In case anyone's wondering, they've noticed.

LET ME EXPLAIN...

Then, when we do talk, a second lampooned tendency with a kernel of truth shows itself: that is, to offer a solution when not asked for one, for which we supposedly have a natural gift and a universal mandate. Or to explain to women in the simplest of terms what needs no explanation, referred to as both 'mansplaining' and (more amusingly) 'correctile dysfunction'.

As a term, mansplaining dates from a 2008 essay by Rebecca Solnit entitled: 'Explain Things to Me: Facts Didn't Get in Their Way'. The subtitle is the interesting part; no facts required. Research concludes, after all, that brilliance is a male trait.

We're all – men and women alike – inclined, individually and collectively, to take a half-complete story and add what we think the missing parts may be until it sounds believable.

There's plenty of credible evidence that this really happens. The diagnosis of ailments in others – real or not – is an area in which this often shows itself.

The less complete the story, the wilder the additions often are. *"Have you seen Joan? She's been sweating a lot recently and been off sick a few times. A mate saw it in a film at the weekend, and I reckon it's malaria. Best steer clear."*

So, we like explaining things, and tend to fill in the gaps with whatever seems to fit in order to offer an explanation. Combined, it doesn't bode well for when our partner's menopause arrives. We're all lifehackers now, with a ready-made diagnosis for everything. So, we'll have an explanation for the event, but one that in all probability will *not* be the menopause.

SORRY, WHAT?

Both avoidance and mansplaining actively work against the more important half of conversation: listening. That is, actually taking in what's been said, processing and understanding. If necessary, asking for clarification or more information and taking that in too. Not just asking to indicate interest without having any. It also doesn't mean waiting for our turn to speak.

There's no downside to being a great listener. Most men just haven't worked out yet that being a great listener is incredibly sexy. For the remainder of this chapter where 'talking' is mentioned, for the sake of brevity, it'll be assumed to include active listening too.

GROUND RULES

The simple fact is, men should be able to talk about the menopause with anyone, not just as a necessary response when pushed. There are three aspects for us to be aware of when talking about menopause with women, irrespective of whether the woman in question is menopausal:

- We don't want to be continually nodding and pretending, wondering when we may get to a search engine or AI chatbot to check a few details in case we'd been rumbled. So, there's knowing enough about it to be able to engage. Having a basic grounding is vital. Luckily, this book contains one, so excuses aren't available any longer. If you haven't found it, you just skipped past it: it's the first chapter.
- Then there's understanding the male role. Unless we're a medical doctor – and if we are, unless we've studied the menopause – it's not to offer a solution. We're not engaging to fix, but to understand, listen and offer only what's requested. We must think of discussing the menopause as an amazingly practical way to beneficially rewire our behaviour. If we can master it here, we'll master it everywhere and be the better for it. And yes, others will notice. Because if we err in attempting to understand our

role, we'll soon be told in no uncertain terms to shut the heck up. Menopausal women tend to say it as it is, only worse. As may have already become apparent, the rules of engagement are different from the perimenopause onwards. It's a rollercoaster of discovery.

- It's understanding that the conversation won't be a one-off box-ticking exercise but will be ongoing – for up to a decade and, for some, beyond. To borrow a sometimes-medical expression, we'll be 'on call', 24/7/365 throughout. Yet to set aside any fears of repetition, it won't be the same conversation over and over. As we've established, the subject of the conversation will change as the symptoms and their patterns change. Which, let's face it, will mean that it'll always be interesting, sometimes surprising and often dangerous.

The ground rules established, there are some things we can do to help embed active talking and listening in our relationship with our partner.

🎬 NEIL'S ACTION PLAN

LIVE, TALK AND LEARN

Intentionally avoid judgement. Kate and I have talked about the menopause from when it began till now, when we're writing about talking about it and talking about writing about it. We made it a shared experience. Kate's menopause is now not as ferocious as it once was, yet we're still talking about it.

WHY?

- We'll always be learning. And learning is a good thing. At the outset, I didn't have the benefit of a book that wasn't a medical doorstop to hand; I learned as Kate learned. She would explain to me what was happening, why, what to expect, what she was planning to do about it and what she needed me to do. She would warn me when she was losing control. I wasn't asked my opinion, and I made sure I didn't offer it. In some senses it was a relief, as I didn't have one to give. I had no idea this would be her chosen career thereafter, just that we were trying to understand what was happening and to ensure it didn't impact our lives. I had no idea we'd be writing a book either, until Kate suggested it.

- It's not just about our relationship with our partner. We'll encounter menopausal women everywhere in our life. So, learning to listen and talk about it at home will stand us in good stead. I began thinking during the early stages of Kate's symptoms about the working relationships that may have been overshadowed by the menopause, and I must admit I felt embarrassed at what incorrect conclusions I may have drawn at the time. I'm now sensitive to what may be occurring. Which also means I don't draw conclusions. Just as an emotional reaction may be due to the menopause, it may not be.

GAUGE

We have to remain sensitive to when and how our partner may wish to talk about her menopause – and on occasion, be the one to take the initiative. While, as we just mentioned, we're avoiding judgment, here timing is a matter of judgement.

WHY?

- If we think, as men, that we're struggling to talk about menopause, then women are too, but to a far greater degree. As we covered in the previous chapter, we must remain aware of the historical and social context, the scale of negative perceptions they have to overcome in even beginning to talk. As men, there's nothing natural in our lives that compares, we have no direct experience to draw on. "I know how you must feel" will never apply.

- Although awkward, if the conversation just isn't happening, we may be required to gauge the moment and carefully raise the subject. We must start the conversation with our partner when it may not be welcome and maintain it when we'd really rather it be dismissed. As may be apparent, we've moved on quite a bit from where we were at the start of this chapter. It's got a bit trickier than just being prepared to have a chat about our partner's sweats occasionally and offer a word of empathetic comfort.

ADAPT

We need to hone the art of adapting how we talk and listen. Even if we're already good at it. What works today may not work tomorrow.

WHY?

- The old rules and boundaries won't apply. There's no shying away from the fact that the conversation is likely to be rocky at times. Jokes that are personal to us both, once funny, may suddenly become incendiary if they hit a nerve. Spoiler alert: it'll seem like there are more 'nerves' to hit too. Our partner's levels of tolerance may vary from low to impossibly low. What may feel to us like a good time to talk may turn out to be the worst choice we ever made to raise a subject.

- There will never be a return to 'normal', as in post-menopause it'll be different again. That's not to say we can't draw on what once worked for us both. The menopause is a time for us to get used to a new way of talking and listening together. One characterised by more time for, and a deeper understanding of, one another.

RECONCILE

If we find ourselves frustrated, stuck, shut down, feeling that we can't win – we must simply remind ourselves which one of us is having the menopause.

WHY?

- We're not experiencing the symptoms and their consequences. And it's worth stating, 'winning' has no part to play: we're in it together. At which point the chiselled, brooding man of few words from the big screen may instead become the interested, engaged and responsive type who can make a positive difference to the women around them. A real hero.

- The by-product of honing the art of conversation during the menopause, for both parties in a relationship and many parties in the wider world of work and social life, is that we all get better at talking. If we can talk about the menopause and it makes a difference, we can talk about nearly anything else with sensitivity, skill and ease. It can't be stressed enough, therefore, that there's absolutely *no compromise on masculinity* by being able to do so.

○ ○ ○

That this chapter is located early in this book isn't an accident. We'll keep coming back to its key message: talking with our partner is essential. If we're unable to talk to one another through the menopause then we can forget the rest, give up now, hide or check out. We must be prepared to talk for both our sakes – and for the health, survival and growth of the relationship. If we don't, our partner won't want us around, because they'll think we're useless. And they'll be absolutely right.

4

EXPECTATIONS

The menopause will change a woman biologically and emotionally. It can therefore alter the expectations she has of herself, of her partner and those her partner has of her, all of which will have implications for the relationship.

EXPECTATIONS: KATE

CAN WE HAVE IT ALL?

As women, we juggle multiple expectations from all directions. Overall, we're meant to be:

- Well-behaved yet challenging
- Compliant yet forceful

- Deferential yet successful
- Predictable yet risk-taking
- Youthful but ageing gracefully

At home we're supposed to be:

- Obedient wives (which means biddable, even if not married)
- Off-duty catwalk models
- Insatiable sex kittens
- Award-winning chefs
- Attentive hosts
- Caring mothers and daughters
- There for everyone, all the time
- Brilliant at just about everything
- All the above at the same time

You've ticked them all, right? Is there any wonder women struggle to have it all, if that's what 'all' entails?

Forming expectations is human. We use expectations as a scale to assess ourselves and others. They're culturally embedded. We're all responsible for their formation and for their permanence.

This is a tricky but important chapter, as it sets the scene for much of what will happen in our relationship during the menopause. The easiest way to think of the three types of expectation we'll consider is: self, self to partner, partner to self. As the list above suggests, we've started with ourselves.

Society forms expectations of us as women, which we sub-consciously take on board and harden into expectations of ourselves. A constant need to compare ourselves to others is a spiky stick we beat ourselves with daily.

But we can't have it all. Not even those who appear to, whatever their social media feeds would have us believe. At least not without an army of skilled helpers and an evergreen money tree to fund them. We're all somewhere on a sliding scale ranging from success to failure at any point throughout our lives, and on any given day, too. In trying to manage our quite ridiculous expectation of ourselves something must give, and it's usually our wellbeing.

IF IT WASN'T DIFFICULT ENOUGH...

Then there are the expectations we'll have of our partner, and the expectations they'll have of us. Every relationship we have is based on expected behaviour, both ways. We're creatures of habit and seekers of patterns, because they make our lives simple, comfortable and easy to navigate. And so we use observation and experience of past behaviour to predict how others will react in certain situations. We'll then adjust our behaviour towards them accordingly.

For example, if we know a friend becomes visibly irritated when we're vague or non-committal, we'll try to be direct and decisive in their company. We'll probably have given up trying to change them, or maybe never even mentioned it to them. Sometimes we're aware that we're doing this, sometimes not; it's automatic.

All this was before we got to our menopause. It ramps everything up another league in three ways, which may or may not be recognisable, by:

- Impacting our expectations of ourselves, removing our ability to even remember the things we're supposed to be amazing at (helpfully, you'll have the list in this chapter to refer to) – and most certainly removing our ability to be amazing at them (if we once thought we were).
- Impacting our ability to meet the expectations others will have of us.
- Considerably changing our expectations of how others should behave towards us.

In short, we're going to be different, and we'll want others to be different.

CHANGING DYNAMICS

Initially, when the menopause arrives, we'll try and carry on regardless.

Most of us won't have drifted to this point in our lives on clouds of fortune. We'll have faced adversity, won some battles and lost others.

Anxiety, however, is a common symptom of the menopause,

and one that we're only just starting to discuss. For many it's a symptom that creeps in under darkness and wriggles its way into every experience, making us question ourselves – what we can and can't do, should and shouldn't do – and the attitudes and motivations of those around us.

Depression, anxiety's more sinister cousin, is far more common in women than public discussion recognises. Suicide rates among women are at their highest during the menopause years due to complex issues around mental, physical and financial wellbeing, as well as the availability of appropriate and effective support. It's important therefore to take it seriously. If it feels darker than a mere dip in the road, it's time to stop expecting ourselves to quickly re-emerge.

FLUSH TO CRUSH

Experiences during the early years of my menopause show how all three expectations can be impacted.

My hot flushes were horrific. I would sweat profusely and turn bright red. I'd look like I'd just run a marathon in full makeup, which had slid down my face. My primitive brain would switch off any thought other than "I am so hot I don't know what to do".

If I was at an evening social event, I knew I'd have at least six hot flushes throughout. Yet I always felt incredibly ill prepared when they occurred, even though I knew they would.

The expectation of others was that if I was there, my

behaviour and responses would, or should, be predictable. The Kate they knew. When a hot flush began, people would look a little unnerved and would start to edge away. *I wasn't the Kate they knew*. Or if they didn't know me, I wasn't behaving within the acceptable norms for the type of person they assumed I was. I'd frantically reach for anything I could flap in front of my face. I even used a ceramic plate once – needs must.

I would mumble that I was sorry, that it was my menopause, and that it would pass. As I learned far too slowly, feebly flapping, meekly apologising and sweating rivers never persuades anyone that we're in control.

They'd 'see' someone over the other side of the room that they simply *had* to talk to and exit quickly. Even if that someone didn't exist. Or I'd be summarily dismissed by women who hadn't had the same experience as me, or had but weren't owning up to it. I felt crushed, small and insignificant. The urge to leave was as much as I could contain. You can imagine what that did to my self-esteem and anxiety levels.

Interestingly, however, those that slipped away often discreetly returned to me a short while later to request more information, either for themselves or their partner, maybe even 'asking for a friend'. I assumed that they were managing their expectation that they wouldn't have an experience like mine. Or respond in the way that I did. All the while crossing their fingers, toes and everything else.

INTO THE SHADOWS, AGAIN

It was another example of how the menopause sits below society's surface, present but denied, discussed in private or in hushed tones.

The urge to stand on a table and shout it at the top of my voice was in the long queue of things I wanted to do but didn't. Instead, I often chose to leave quietly or sob uncontrollably in the toilet. Once your mascara has kissed goodbye to your eyes and said hello to your cheeks through sweating, crying no longer holds the same fear.

If Neil was with me at such an event, however, he was oblivious to how I was feeling. This was incredibly hard. I wanted him to step in and support me – *not save me* – but he didn't. He didn't see me crumple because I was desperately trying not to let it show, and he wasn't looking out for it. He had his expectations of me. I was the Kate he knew, as there were no obvious indicators to the contrary other than sweating, which had quickly become part of our lives.

I'd always dealt with awkward situations capably. I was shy but socially comfortable, able to create conversation and invite openness. Neil's expectation of me was that, even with the menopause, I'd be fine, unless I specifically asked for help. This was a fair assumption, as it was how we managed other areas of our life. Faced with any kind of challenge we'd talk about it, agree what we'd each do and get on with it. If that didn't work, one of us flagged it and made an alternative suggestion.

This wasn't happening. I wasn't talking about it. Even though I was effectively hiding it while crying in the ladies' toilet, I expected him to know. Neil meanwhile wasn't looking out for it and didn't recognise that he was meant to.

My response was in no way reasonable. It made me angry, and at times fairly unpleasant. I bottled it up until the resentment got too much and, sometime later, like Vesuvius, I exploded, and shouted at him. Obviously not the best approach.

The warning here is that not managing our expectations of one another through the menopause can cause a corrosive resentment in a relationship. The menopause can be a downward spiral.

There are three actions we can take in resetting our expectations during the menopause, directly related to the trinity of: self, self to partner, and partner to self.

🎬 KATE'S ACTION PLAN

RESET THE EXPECTATION OF OURSELVES

We must take the pressure off ourselves during the menopause. We've nothing to say sorry for. This is a natural part of life. Every woman will have a menopause. And there's no list of attributes we must be striving for – we've enough to be dealing with.

WHY?

- The pressure we place ourselves under is a destructive waste of energy. We have to stop being overly critical of ourselves. The menopause has a way of making us feel isolated, as though we're the only one in the world experiencing this, or worse, the only one not managing to stay on top of it. We berate ourselves for the effect our symptoms have on us and our inability to regain control. That our symptoms are effectively consuming who we are, making us withdraw to the shadows. The reality is we haven't created this situation, but we can create a way out.

- We must do this to help ourselves literally stand up, feel our power and stop apologising. Sensing this was happening to me, I could feel myself shout out: "not bloody likely, I am *not* my menopause!" It drove me to straighten myself and stare the beast down. It's amazing how much better we feel when we step into the power of our physicality.

HELP OUR PARTNER RESET THEIR EXPECTATION OF US

As we covered in the previous chapter, we need to let our partner know what's happening and what we need. The sooner the better. We can't wait for them to work it out. The imperative is with us. We should also be prepared for several conversations, not just one. And we shouldn't leave it on a sticky note on the fridge for when they get home.

WHY?

- If we're a confident and able woman, giving out the 'I can cope' signals to our partner, drifting swan-like past them while beneath the surface paddling frantically, manically holding on to our composure, they're going to take it as the norm. After all, that's the way we've always been and we've always managed, until this point.

- It's not for us to do everything within our power to continue to function emotionally and physically as we once did for our partner's benefit, to meet their expectations of us. On the contrary, it's for them to understand the menopause, what we're going through and reset with us. It's the same with others close to us, whether family or friends.

RESET OUR EXPECTATION OF OUR PARTNER

We'll have a reasonable expectation of how open, under-standing and practical our partner may be as the menopause arrives. Hopefully, if the relationship is thriving, it'll be (mostly) positive. Yet we must also recognise that they're about to see us change, which won't be easy for them. At times, they may be challenged by it. We'll need to allow them to be vulnerable too. With many aspects of our partner's support during the menopause, there's little heroic about it. Which is why, as covered in the 'Talking' chapter, we'll have to set out what might happen, what the triggers for intervention by them may be, and the potential nature and frequency of that intervention. Importantly, too, when we need them to simply observe and be ready in case. Just to be there.

WHY?

- There's a big difference between our partner supporting and saving us. 'Saving' is about them stepping in and taking over, which can be coercive, uncomfortable and rather embarrassing. We don't need that. He's not our knight on a steed, nor are we a defenceless and helpless maiden. We can leave that to the major studios – they have a much bigger budget. If Neil had jumped in every time someone said something to me about the menopause, it would have been a thankless full-time job for him and tedious for us both.

- There's a delicate balance between allowing our partner to adjust, respecting their struggle in seeing us in difficulty and our needing to be a counsellor. We need to see that they are understanding the menopause, its effect on us and adapting.

- Where there are signs that our partner is unprepared to invest that small amount of time and energy required to adjust with us, we must question whether there's a future in the relationship. If our partner says, "I didn't sign up for this" – neither did we!

- The menopause means we'll have neither the patience nor inclination to hang on to a relationship that's breaking, even if we fear being alone. In many respects, acknowledging that we can take such a decision offers an early insight into how we'll be in our post-menopause and second-phase years.

○ ○ ○

During the menopause, as the symptoms change in nature and severity, we'll be continually resetting the expectations we have of ourselves and others, and they have of us. As with almost everything during the menopause, expectations are never fixed. The nature and level of that adjustment is something we can control.

EXPECTATIONS: NEIL

WE'VE GOT THIS – HAVEN'T WE?

When our partner's menopause arrives, there'll be an expectation of how we'll be, based on a heady mix of how we've been with our partner in any number of situations before, and society's depiction of men in challenging situations.
Either:

- We'll be utterly crap. And honestly, what's the point in even trying to get us to understand? It's a total waste of time. We'll make a chocolate teapot look like a handy addition to any kitchen; or
- We'll get it instantly, understand the menopause for what it is and will become, and we'll be limitlessly and instinctively helpful and supportive throughout.

Or, quite possibly, over time, a combination of the two. But a combination isn't easy to either imagine or describe. It certainly doesn't make for a good sit-com script.

Being honest with ourselves about how we react to challenging situations can be tricky, if we even consciously consider it at all. We of course might actually be amazing, whether we're aware of it or not. But we'll probably have a mixed record, dragged down at times by bad luck (obviously) and the underperformance of others (inevitably). It would be a rare man to contentedly award himself no points at all, with no plan to do better next time – and a rare woman to tolerate him.

Our partner's expectation of us will veer towards one of these extremes too. They'll have the examples as evidence, if needed. If the expectation isn't looking too rosy for us, we'll deploy the same reasoning we used with ourselves to head off any negativity: we'd have been better if it wasn't for [insert reason].

So, while we'll laugh at the hilarious portrayals of hapless men on screen, we'll back ourselves to be capable, and we'll expect our partner to back us too.

However, we shouldn't underestimate the difficulty of seeing our partner go through the menopause, particularly if they're one of the quarter of women for whom it's awful. It's only natural that we're going to feel helpless, some or all the time, seeing someone we love suffer and having no solutions to offer.

THEY'VE GOT THIS – HAVEN'T THEY?

We'll have an expectation, too, of how our partner will deal with their menopause. It'll determine our estimate of how much support we may need to give.

We'll have seen if they're the tough-it-out type or the crumble-hopelessly variety from what they'll have been through before. We'll expect them to follow their normal path that will – as with their expectation of us – fill us with either confidence or dread.

But the unique, relentless and changeable nature of the menopause can alter how our partner responds in ways we – and they – may not have seen before. Initial toughness may be slowly yet irreversibly eroded, leading to a long, slow and barely noticeable surrender. Or early submission to the symptoms may be thrown off by the mustering of a deep determination to fight back. Or, over time, both.

The truth is, at the outset, even though neither of us will know, we'll more than likely be confident, because we'll have observed, or just have a sense, that women seem inherently able to handle what life throws at them. Added to which, with increased (but still inadequate) coverage of the menopause in the media, that as an outcome, all women are now better prepared.

As the symptoms reveal themselves, therefore, we'll be backing our brilliance and our partner's resilience. Which will, of course, in all probability be entirely wrong. So, where are these expectations coming from?

NOTHING TO SEE HERE...

Much of what we expect of our partner, they of us and we of ourselves, isn't the result of conscious thought. It's created by the lens through which we all view the world.

Our world view is built from the widest possible collection of personal and societal influences during our life. It's being shaped every single day like a clay pot on a wheel. These influences include every aspect of the universal loading in favour of (white) men to which we're exposed from our earliest years, and solidifies as we grow up.

In the formation of our world view, as men, our understanding of what it means to be a woman is minimal. We barely think about what a woman must face. As we don't constantly swim against a tide of judgment and bias, we're often unaware of the effort it takes women to battle it all their lives, at every turn.

Take the physical and emotional effects of around thirty years of the menstrual cycle. We might see it as a mere inconvenience (to us, mainly). Similarly, we can have no idea of how carrying a baby for nine months and then delivering it – especially a natural birth – might feel. We may empathise, ask questions or do some research, but we can't know what it's like.

In a much-research area of biology, it's recognised that, while women overall have a lower pain threshold than men, their life experiences better prepare them for handling it. Despite that, it's been proven that doctors take reports of pain more seriously from men than from women. Even in the consulting room it's stacked against women.

It's no surprise therefore that when our partner's menopause arrives, as a man we may just see it as another inevitable and unavoidable event in a lifelong series for them. They'll just deal with it. A view, unfortunately, advanced by some female commentators who had an easy menopause, or a menopause they're not prepared to admit was difficult.

Meanwhile, we're focused on whether hair implants might be a good move.

The reality, of course, isn't anywhere near as simple as our opening options suggested. Over time together, we'll have forged roles with which the other is generally happy. We become accustomed to things our partner is capable of handling on their own, to knowing where our assistance or involvement is necessary. It's reassuringly predictable, leaving time for more interesting stuff.

Essentially, we're expecting us to do what we've always done. Which, of course, we won't. With the menopause, our expectations of one another will therefore, to a huge degree, start to form again from scratch.

MESSING UP

In the process of writing this book, Kate relayed a situation to me with which I was rather horrified when I realised I royally messed up.

Some friends were at our house, and in conversation Kate raised her extremely difficult menopause experience. Both responded with a wave of the hand, brushing off like a fruit fly a matter that they claimed made no difference to their lives. As though they were in disbelief of Kate's experience.

I expected Kate to be able to handle this situation as she would always do with difficult conversations. She's incredibly good at them. But it transpired she needed my intervention, to support her description of her experience, yet it didn't come. She thought I would, because in most matters I was always keen to help and support. I'd misjudged. I expected her to handle it, she expected me to intervene, neither of which happened. Having talked it out, I now know, and I'm ready. But it took a lot of time, upset and emotion to get there.

We need to note that our partner's menopause isn't a test of our character or resolve, a battle of wills, a struggle against a foe that's always one step ahead of us. And so, if we're wondering what new forms of guile, strength and resilience we'll need to acquire for the menopausal struggle, that would be the wrong way entirely to view the situation.

As the general gist of this book may have already revealed though, we'll have some work ahead. It's not all down to our partner, while we look on. Or look away. Here's what we can do.

🎬 NEIL'S ACTION PLAN

ACKNOWLEDGE VULNERABILITY

We must recognise, understand and then acknowledge our own vulnerability – however capable we may have been in the past. Feeling vulnerable is not a failure on our part, it's entirely natural. We don't need to 'man up' as we mentioned in the 'Talking' chapter, even if our partner expects a more measured or stoical response from us initially. Similarly, us doing the same for our partner's vulnerability is a vital early step, however capable *they've* been in the past, as things are happening to them that they possibly don't understand or over which they feel they're not in control. All of which means talking about it, and agreeing how we can both take small steps to build confidence, individually and together.

WHY?

- We're both entirely permitted to have feelings and to be free to talk about them, or we'll be storing up resentment for the future when unrealistic expectations of one another aren't met.
- As the arrival of the menopause for our partner will most likely be incremental, rather than announcing itself dramatically with ticker tape and trumpets, our vulnerability may sneak in under the door too. We'll need heightened self-awareness, so we're attuned to the changes

in our emotional state. Men are encouraged to perform regular physical checks on themselves to look for signs of a problem – this is no different.

LEARN TO ADJUST

This is a new phase in our life, and our life together, that requires us to adjust all our existing expectations of our partner and ourselves. It'll be a continuous process. Which means we must want to do it, do it and keep doing it. It can be tough, especially where something's worked for us for some time. From here, there are no fixed positions.

WHY?

- Where we don't know what we don't know, we can't plan – we must prepare. Which is about mindset and attitude, two things we can consciously choose. This can't be stressed enough. It's not down to anyone else.
- Our partner needs to see that we're connected with them. We must not only adjust, therefore, but show signs that we're adjusting our behaviour and responses. Small gestures count just as much as bigger ones. This isn't an exercise in PR while seeing what we can get away with.
- In adjusting, we'll probably have to take some 'I knew you'd [insert pathetic contribution]' on the chin at some point, as our partner's assessment of our efforts will be shaped by her emotional state at the time of opening both barrels

on us. But it's part of the process, and not something that should deter us.

- Caution is needed – this doesn't call for an instant 'transformation', throwing away everything we once knew and starting again. The seeds of successful change always lie in the present, as some things will always be working. A totally reinvented 'brave new us' is just as likely to goof it up as the pre-menopausal version.

REDEFINE UNDERSTANDING

In an environment where expectations are forming and reforming, we'll need to replace our instinctive pursuit of balance in our relationship with understanding.

WHY?

- We're taught that successful relationships are about give and take, making an equal contribution over time, always returning to a place of reasonableness. We'll likely have an individual and shared expectation of what being 'reasonable' means. But the menopause doesn't recognise a calm and considered point at which we can set aside every bias, prejudice, emotion and agenda to make a suitable judgment in each situation. At the time of the menopause, that comfortable place becomes more a Lost Property office.
- While we'll both need to show understanding, as partners *we'll* need to show it more. If that brings a frown, think

of what an arse we can be when we feel aggrieved over nothing much at all. In redefining understanding, our self-awareness will require sharpening for the long haul. Which is no bad thing.

o o o

The menopause is an opportunity to explore a closer alignment of our shared expectations and our expectations of one another, as a means both of managing the challenges of the menopause and as preparation for when it's over. It's a mutual learning experience, and one we're well advised from here to see as a worthwhile lifetime's pursuit. Many of the skills and attributes we develop as a partner to a menopausal woman will be useable elsewhere in our life. We have the potential to meet the expectations of our partner *and* emerge a better person.

5

LIFESTYLE

Menopausal symptoms – physical and emotional – may call for lifestyle changes to alleviate them. The changes needed may impact the relationship.

LIFESTYLE: KATE

FACING UP

This must be one of the most difficult chapters to write. Not because there's little to say, but because there's so much to say and none of it's easy.

It's not easy because as women we're incredibly sensitive about so much that this chapter includes. There are some clear choices we can make at this point in life. Should we decide to make them, we're not only looking after ourselves today, but we're also defining how we'll live our lives during our second phase. This is the shiny prize at the end of all of this – a healthy body that enables us to do all the fun things we want to do.

Changing how we view the complex tangle of consumption, excess, denial, craving and reward has, for most of us, been a lifelong tussle.

In our late 30s to early 40s, as we approach our menopause, we're probably still feeling invincible. After all, we're nothing like all those images we see of elderly menopausal ladies, as discussed in the 'Perceptions' chapter: we've still got youth (sort of) and energy (mostly) on our side. But the truth is that during our menopause years we'll enter the zone where risks to our overall health increase. This applies to our partner at this age as well.

Some of the suggestions in this chapter may feel like a step too far, others not far enough. But for those struggling with menopausal symptoms, these changes can lead to regaining much-needed control.

This is one area where a profound difference can be made that will positively impact every symptom together with general wellbeing. Best of all, it's possible to start right now.

In this chapter are the lessons I learnt. They were incredibly difficult. But however tough it was, it was never as bad as facing how I felt about myself at the point I decided to do something about it. This advice is offered to you as one woman to another, without judgment. It's up to you what happens next.

DAWNING REALISATION

As I progressed through my perimenopause, then menopause and into post-menopause, I seemed to change both on the inside and the outside. By the time I hit 50, I wasn't sleeping, I was miserable and eating everything in the name of comfort. I had piled on 18 kilos and there was no sign of it slowing or stopping.

I was deceiving myself that I was exercising. I wasn't.

The swimming pool was too far away – ten minutes' drive. The gym was just wrong. All the local exercise classes seemed to revolve around jumping up and down, which after having two natural births was out of the question: no number of pads or leak-free pants was ever going to be enough. I hated myself and what I'd become. Things had to change, and I was the only one who could make it happen.

WE CAN'T LIE TO OUR BODY

I should say, before perimenopause, I spent at least fifteen years of my life partying like it was 1999.

I bought into the ladette culture of my youth, hook, line, sinker and hangover. I met my girlfriends after work. I started with pints and then migrated to wine and then to champagne (or cheaper versions, depending on funds). I swayed my way home. It felt part of who I was. Typically, I loved the doing, but not so much the feeling the next day. The problem was, and is, that the next day has got more and more agonising over the years, to the point where it now begins before the last drink is finished.

My mum has severe osteoporosis, and I've seen first-hand how devastating and life-limiting it can be. I went to have my routine bone scan (DEXA) approximately four years ago. The nurse who did the scan looked at the results and with a frown asked me how many units of alcohol a week I was drinking. After a quick recall of the government-recommended limit, I lied and said sixteen. Who doesn't? She gave me a long hard stare as though she was surfacing that very lie and said, "It should be no more than ten." I think I shrieked; I can't be sure. But what I can say is that when the report arrived with the news that my osteopenia (the precondition to osteoporosis) had severely worsened, all I could hear were her words.

Everything changed in that moment.

The drinking from then on has been kept to within ten units a week, the equivalent of a bottle of wine. Well, mostly.

This event coincided with the realisation that 98 per cent of my wardrobe no longer fitted. Buttons popped and zips wouldn't do up. The slow incremental change to my body could no longer be ignored. I was stressed and desperate.

I had to make some wellbeing decisions for myself.

THE TIPPING POINT

In my experience, from speaking to menopausal women all day every day, most of us arrive at the point during the menopause when we know we must make changes. There are multiple drivers, and no two women are the same, but there are common threads. They include:

- Weight gain or change in body shape
- Ill health
- Symptom management
- A life event (positive or negative)
- To rescue their self-esteem

Let's talk about the most sensitive subject in that list first.

Weight gain or change in body shape has its hooks into our health and self-esteem. For me, it was soul-destroying to see the scales continually nudging upwards, no matter what I did. There's a reason for this, and it's not that the scales were broken. As our ovaries decide it's all too much like hard work to keep producing oestrogen due to the dwindling number of eggs, our bodies look elsewhere for help. After all, we've got rather dependent on these chemicals and don't want to face life without them. The fat in our body is good at producing oestrogen and the fat around our middle is very, very good at it. Essentially, our bodies are actively seeking to put weight on in this area to boost the supply of oestrogen. This can have negative consequences.

I know that I could have taken the view that there was more of me for Neil to love, but that didn't help me or make me love me. It's important to note, at no point did Neil mention my weight or for that matter seem to notice my body had changed. This was about me.

The principal downside of weight gain, especially when it gets out of hand, is it makes us more prone to numerous cancers – and if things do get out of hand, more susceptible to type 2 diabetes and heart disease. There's no point deceiving ourselves, these are the risks, and we need to choose how we respond to them. Because it's a choice.

I need to say at this juncture, if you're living with obesity and have got to the point where you'd like to lose weight, I wholeheartedly applaud you. I also recommend you ask your doctor for support to address the yo-yoing that many in this situation experience. Don't give up, there's so much to benefit from.

FINDING THE FUN

Exercise must go hand in hand with any change in what we eat and drink. Without it, we're trying to win the race while relaxing in the armchair. Literally. Movement is the gift that keeps on giving. It releases our feel-good hormones, benefits our body and importantly helps with our mental health. But to do this we must find something we like doing so much that we keep going back for more.

For my part, getting to the pool seemed like too much effort.

I needed a new exercise. One that was practical, with no reason not to do it. I'm incredibly resolute once I've decided. But if it's something I don't want to do or am not particularly bothered about, I'll prevaricate. I know I'm not alone in this.

I tried power-walking, which always ended up more walk, less power. I tried the gym, which I've persisted with but still don't like, but I do it for strength, muscle retention and balance. So, I turned to running. At this point I couldn't run at all. I hurt all over and I gasped for air as I tried to flag down the number 52 bus. But it was free and accessible – sort of – just outside my front door.

I downloaded a running app onto my phone, listened to the motivating celebrity voices, put my low-fashion trainers on and stepped outside with the trepidation of a newbie. If you're wondering if I found out that I was a natural, sadly not. The first three months were agony, quite literally. My body was royally annoyed with me for not doing it sooner and for letting things get so out of hand. I got numerous injuries and had to invest in a decent sports bra and trainers. But I'd decided this was my exercise, and I wasn't giving up. Without question, running got me (and my family) through the pandemic. It's now an intrinsic part of me, and I need it, both for my physical and mental wellbeing.

As can be imagined, there's a lot we can potentially do for or wellbeing. Essentially, I'll talk about a combination of what we eat and drink, and exercise. We cover sleep in the later chapter on 'Night and Day', albeit managing the above can make a significant contribution to better sleep. Lastly our mental health underpins everything – it'll be covered in the 'Moods' chapter, along with stress.

▶ KATE'S ACTION PLAN

CUT IT OUT

We can help ourselves today by cutting out the consumption of several things. Most won't be a surprise. Decisive action puts us in the driving seat and that feels bloody brilliant during the menopause, a time when there seems very little control to be had. We shouldn't underestimate the contribution this alone can make.

WHY?

- Sugar is incredibly addictive and bad for almost every part of our body; once it's in our system, most of us crave it. It's squeezed into almost every processed food available. If we're cutting it out, we simply must go cold turkey. We'll likely not be able to manage a steadily declining level because it's too tempting to just have one square of chocolate; we'll inevitably finish the whole bar.
- Nutritionists could probably fill an entire book with reasons why we should avoid processed and fast foods. Not least because they mess with our complex hormonal balance. I'm not a nutritionist; I'll simply say food needn't

be complicated, but it does have to be nutritious. Which, for the avoidance of doubt, most ultra-processed and fast food are not. We can put the 'ready meal' back where it came from and drive past the drive-through.

- Caffeine can stimulate hot flushes, raise anxiety and stress, and worsen insomnia among other things, all major issues during the menopause. It's present in coffee, tea and some fizzy drinks. Again, it's addictive. Substitutes are available and can work. I had to switch to a maximum of two decafs a day, a massive reduction on the six or seven caffeinated coffees I was used to.

- We've already mentioned alcohol, but we'll do so again. It impacts the vitamin and mineral absorption into our bones and is increasingly difficult to process. Plus, many alcoholic drinks are loaded with sugar. We must cut down or cut it out. A useful starter is to always have at least three consecutive days in a week without alcohol at all, then reduce consumption on drinking days. On a drinking day, making the first one alcohol-free helps with the craving. Alcohol-free substitutes have come a long way in recent years.

- If there's anyone out there still smoking, do whatever it takes to stop. Primarily in this instance because smoking is a risk factor in the development of osteoporosis. Vaping is being touted as the 'less harmful' answer to smoking. It's such a new phenomenon that we can't know or predict the long-term effects. What we do know is that the levels of nicotine are highly addictive. Stop this too.

ADD IT BACK

It's not all about reduction and abstinence. There are things we need to add back, too, to help with menopausal symptoms, including water, fruit and vegetables, and vitamin D. They may not seem as exciting as a doughnut and a mocha-choca-latte, syrup and extra whipped cream with sprinkles, but this is a change in thinking as well as behaving. Choosing to do this demonstrates to ourselves as well as others that our wellbeing is primary.

WHY?

- Water flushes out toxins and old used hormones, like adrenalin and cortisol, that hang around our body doing the circuit until we pee them out. The body needs at least two litres (3.5 pints) a day. If we have hot flushes and/or night sweats, more water is a no-brainer. I remember sitting at a skincare stand in a department store and the assistant took one look at my skin and said: "you're massively dehydrated, you need to drink more water". I was mortified. The benefits are far-reaching.

- We need to 'eat a rainbow' – not in that woo-woo unicorn kind of way, but in the manner of fruit and veg. Fresh produce of all colours provides us with nutrients, fibre and some sweetness if we're craving it. Amazingly, gorgeous strawberries and raspberries are low in sugar, as are apples, which are also full of fibre. The more exotic papaya fits into the low-sugar category as well. But mango, bananas, grapes, cherries and figs are all on the high-sugar list and should be eaten sparingly. This is a shame as I can eat a punnet of cherries in one sitting.

- Vitamin D received a great deal of attention during the Covid-19 pandemic as we started to understand its importance for our immune system, and how deficient in it most of us are. During the menopause, our bone production accelerates and our body struggles to provide enough nutrients to support the process, causing our bone density to decrease. We don't notice it until we fall and break a wrist or a hip. Vitamin D, calcium and magnesium supplements can help (as always, seek professional advice first), along with load-bearing exercise: a walk in the park qualifies, as does dancing in the kitchen.

CHEERLEADERS (PART 1)

We must get our partner involved (kids as well if we have them), when we're changing the way we eat and drink. Even the most focused among us would struggle if our favourite indulgence was being joyfully consumed in front of us.

WHY?

- Not bringing our close family along often puts too much temptation in our way. I must give Neil full credit here. As the cook in the house, he's always supported me in the numerous changes I've made to my – and ultimately his and our kids' – diets. I always say why I want to do it, and why extracting certain things and replacing them with others is a better way of being. We talk it through, and he generally goes along with it. In the beginning, I couldn't be at the table if they had a pudding. It was too much of a temptation. But that subsided as the needle on the scales started to drop and I began to feel good about myself. We do have biscuits and chocolate in our house, but we've learned to see them as treats, not the norm.

• We'll need our partner to help us over the occasional hurdle and to stop us from regressing, however stroppy about it we may get. *And we will get stroppy.* I've always given Neil permission to hold me to my initiative in case I fall off the wagon, so to speak. I admit this is hard, but for me it's part of the deal. It also shows our partner our commitment to change and what they need to do to mirror it. This must be a partnership, otherwise we're defining an end before it's even begun.

GET MOVING!

The other half of the initiative is exercise. We need to be honest with ourselves. We all know we should exercise, but to do it we need to find something we enjoy, or at least can manage. Of course, this must be reasonable as some of us have physical limitations or disabilities, as well as other constraints, including finances and time. We can only do what we can do, but doing it is what counts.

WHY?

- The advantages are compelling. Exercise helps us feel better about ourselves, increases our self-esteem, confidence and energy. It helps us sleep, maintains and builds muscle and if it's load-bearing, helps with our bone density. It can also boost our libido. The list goes on.

- Whatever we choose, we must keep doing it regularly – preferably like clockwork – for a minimum of three months. Giving up helps no one, least of all us.

- The repetition creates a useful routine, which gives us the feeling of being in control. It does, of course, require that we stick to it – but when we do, it becomes habitual. Life can get in the way, but we need to commit to ourselves that should we miss our prearranged exercise once, we won't let it happen twice or the habit will quickly begin to unravel.

- It's worth noting, this isn't just a menopause-related initiative. The menopause-managing benefits can be considerable, and if we create new habits they'll last well beyond this phase of life.

CHEERLEADERS (PART 2)

No prizes for guessing that we need to involve our partner (and kids if we have them) with exercise, too. For many of us this will be a marked change. We must be clear. We must define what we're going to do in detail and make it known to those at home. We need to pin it on the wall. This will help us understand what's down to us, and what support we need from them. This must be non-negotiable, or disagreements and resentment will creep in.

WHY?

- As I fell gasping through the door with a face like a beetroot on fire after a lap of the local park, I needed Neil to be my supporter. If he hadn't or, worse, had been dismissive or obstructive, it would've been difficult to continue with the running or could have created a rift between us. If our partner doesn't commit to exercise, there's a danger that we'll grow apart. This goes both ways. If one of us commits and starts to feel good about ourselves, while the other sits on the sofa with a packet of self-pity biscuits, there's a danger we'll become different people. Or perhaps simply different-sized people.

- Joint exercise is a relationship-builder, at a time during the menopause where demonstrations of togetherness are needed. Neil and I talk about running and what might make us better runners. We're also extremely competitive. I'd heard the phrase 'couples who [insert whatever sport you do] together, stay together'. I always thought this was nonsense, but recently Neil was injured and stopped running. It looked like it might be permanent. I was stunned that my own drive to run took a significant dip without the competition. He recovered and things returned to normal. The impact of doing this together can't be underestimated.

- This isn't just about the menopause: we're teaching our kids, if we have them, the benefits of an active lifestyle. Through our initiatives, exercise has become a feature of our whole family's life.

o o o

Health is something we can't buy, but can invest in. Lifestyle planning and change is an intrinsic part of the menopause experience if we want to gain control. The way we live is our choice, and ours alone. Yet we need to understand in our consideration of lifestyle that even when we gain control, we may still need to allow ourselves to lose it from time to time. This is not meant to be a prison, simply a change in perspective that gives us a massive return on our investment.

LIFESTYLE: NEIL

EGGSHELLS

Our partner's menopause has the potential to affect their health. The physical changes it brings can also potentially impact their self-confidence. There are clear and proven lifestyle changes that can address both. But any conversation we may have publicly about the path to a healthier lifestyle is still paved with eggshells.

Read any article we like about lifestyle, and outside of dubious niche conspiracy websites we'll be unlikely to find any encouraging us to:

- Do less exercise.
- Drink more coffee at all hours of the day.
- Eat more processed and ultra-processed foods.
- Drink more alcohol.
- Sleep with whoever we like, whenever we like, without protection.
- Take up smoking or vaping.
- Check our social notifications on our phone in the small hours when we're too wired to sleep.
- When we feel like letting let our hair down, use a selection of illegal recreational drugs to escape the mundanity of daily life.

As Kate stated, at the time of our partner's menopause years we'll all likely be 'in the zone' where risks to our general health increase. Men begin to be far more susceptible to heart disease from age 45 onwards, and our risk of a stroke doubles every ten years from age 55.

But even by our early 40s, we're still struggling, to a huge extent, with what we see as 'good' and what we see as 'bad'. The things we know are good for us to do or consume we may consider bad for our sanity, the things we know are bad for us we may deem good for our soul.

Our perspective has changed a little in the tech 'start-up' era, with stories of unconventional, eccentric company founders in the full flush of youth carving out lives of puritanical self-denial while making billions on the side. But it can be argued that their tendency to get out of bed before most nightclubs are closed is simply the opposite form of unhinged disregard for the self.

Yoga at 4 a.m., anyone? I didn't think so. There must be a balance available.

MAKE YOUR MIND UP TIME

On this eggshell path, therefore, Kate and I agonised over how we should write this chapter. We went from full-bore shock therapy to embarrassed apology and back again.

But we need to remember that, with exceptions of course, most of us have got a reason for why we're in the state of health we're in right now. For most of us, it's the result of choices we've made and are making every day. There's no point in hiding from those choices.

At times in our life, we may be forced to take tough decisions, with all sorts of physical, mental, spiritual and social consequences. If we're advised to give up or reduce habits or consumption we've been enjoying, we may see the outcome as the removal of all the fun from our lives. Or we may see it as creating different sources of satisfaction and happiness. Probably more of the former, to begin with, until we've tried it.

We may ask at the outset therefore, with some trepidation and rather not wanting to hear the answer: is all of this going to make us boring?

We should say, that for some already making the choices I'll recommend, it may mean almost no lifestyle change at all. It then depends on what's deemed to be boring. Other people when drunk, for example, aren't especially interesting. Only we can make ourselves boring. Let's face it, being interesting all the time is both exhausting and impossible. So perhaps we shouldn't torture ourselves with the worry.

Along with the social challenge, over the longer term the only other potential downsides to being healthier are the time and dedication it requires. I would say financial investment, too, but it's often far cheaper than burning the candle at both ends.

Then throw the menopause into the mix – a life-transforming physical change over which women have little initial control – and suddenly the choices around lifestyle come into sharper focus. For both of us.

ENGAGED OR INVOLVED?

As Kate has described, our partner will at some point need to confront a series of lifestyle choices, the menopause bringing on a trinity of physical and emotional lost control:

- The symptoms we addressed at the start of the book.
- Specific ailments or illnesses brought about by the drop in hormones, such as osteoporosis.
- Progressively negative feelings about herself because of the first two above. The hit to our partner's self-esteem from the menopause can't be stressed enough.

The choices therefore move from being an option to a necessity.

Which will inevitably involve us on a scale from acknowledgement, through cheerleading – what we might call 'engagement' – all the way to full-blown involvement.

When our partner presents us with "I have to…", this often means "*we* have to…". If we imagine it the other way around, we'd probably expect full compliance from our partner and a whole bucketload of sympathy on demand too. It places us in a position where what once may have been optional – to be part of it for the full duration – becomes a necessity.

Just like Kate, I'm a stubborn bugger. So, when Kate pitched the idea that "we're going to have to make some changes around here", I was all in for being part of the plan. I didn't know what the plan was at the time, but I did know that most of the elements would probably make me feel better in the morning, feel better about myself and be better to be with.

The aims all sounded worth pursuing, as if subconsciously I was looking for a reason anyway. At least to begin with. I was also aware that in committing I would at times need to be the one who reminded us of the mission, as asking for change can often be a request to "help me change". With all such initiatives, someone must have this role.

The ability to pursue a healthier lifestyle is, of course, likely to be impacted by personal circumstances. Just as with the menopause itself, it begins with an awareness of what's possible, and how to achieve and maintain it.

Each of the actions we can take with lifestyle is a clear and meaningful signal of our commitment to help our partner through the menopause. My plan considers the same areas as Kate's, but from a different perspective.

🎬 NEIL'S ACTION PLAN

SLOWER FOOD

We must review our dietary choices and adjust what we consume. We must be part of our partner's plan, and plan with them. That means both of us reducing our intake of sugar, salt, saturated fats, processed and ultra-processed foods. I should add that balance in our diet applies to vegetarians and vegans too.

WHY?

- Our partner's ability to control their weight can collapse during the menopause and their fightback begins with what they eat. Which means what we eat – we're going to need to work together on it to make it successful.

- Cooking is cool – hardly anyone thinks it's naff not to know how. If we don't know how, it means learning, alone or together, which in turn means us trying a variety of foods. We can take the lead in research, meal-planning, shopping for food and its preparation. We can make food interesting and meals a time to talk. That includes talking about the learning – what's working, what's not, and what we might do differently.

SLOWER LIFE

We must both be aware of, and manage, the effects of stress on our diet. In fact, on our entire wellbeing. Which means taking steps to identify the causes of stress and avoid or reduce them. Doing so together, and holding ourselves to our commitments, is far easier than trying to do so alone.

WHY?

- Stress reduces the effectiveness of our immune system. By the time of the menopause, neither of us will be spring chickens, and so we'll need this kit to be fully functional. If we're not well, chances are we won't be exercising.
- Stress provokes a need for sugar which then prompts poor sleep which by the morning prompts a need for sugar and increases stress. And so, it goes on. It's an ecosystem of trouble.

SOFTER DRINK

For some men, reducing alcohol is the hardest commitment to make with our partner. Of course, we may each already drink little or no alcohol, in which case we can skip this section. If we do drink, we can't expect our partner to cut down and we not to. To clarify, our target, in the region of 10–12 units, is per week, not per night. We have to start to plan for not exceeding it. If we're not practised in the dull art of counting our units, we need to be, which means knowing how many are in each drink. We need to forget any idea of claiming that the unit limits have no basis in science and so we should ignore them. As with eating, adjusting and moderating our drinking is far easier together than alone.

WHY?

- Alcohol exacerbates many of the symptoms of the menopause, which can cause health problems for our partner. It's as simple as that.
- It'll help us eat better. Alcohol creates cravings for the wrong foods, at the wrong time of day (or night). Three pints after a hard day and all I can see thereafter is a kebab, and it's beautiful. We've all done it. It needs untangling.
- We forget how many calories and how much sugar is contained in alcoholic drinks. For our partner, this can conflict with their desire to eat more healthily. For men, beer bellies are never a good look.

- It'll help us sleep better, which we'll need at this time. We'll come on to the havoc the menopause can wreak after darkness in the chapter on 'Night and Day'.

DEEPER BREATHS

If either of us are smoking, we just need to stop. Now. Stop vaping too. And stop taking anything bought on street corners or under the railway arches.

WHY?

- Do I really need to say? They'll play havoc with a menopause as much as they'll play havoc with life, relationships and a bank balance.

SWEATIER SOCKS

Our partner will need to exercise regularly, and so therefore will we. We'll need to encourage one another from time to time, as it'll be a drain on time and energy, and we'll often have other things we want or need to do. For us both, life can get in the way of our commitment to our body. As Kate and I discovered and as she mentioned in her section, an element of competitiveness always helps. Kate and I can't do anything like this without competing, which has kept us both entirely focused.

WHY?

- Exercise has physical, mental and emotional benefits. For our partner, it's a defence against weight gain, but also important in managing anxiety, self-esteem, mood swings and other mental and emotional effects of menopause. It's a key aspect of regaining control that our partner may seek at this time. We'll get similar benefit, too, if we're struggling with work or personal problems. A sense of control can benefit us both. And help us fight off the moobs.

- To expect our partner to have enough self-discipline to see it through while we look on is unfair. So, assuming we're able, we'll need to get out on the streets, too. Or an equivalent exercise – it doesn't have to be the same. But the commitment needs to be held, progress measured between us. I'd been running for most of my adult life, on and off, so picking it up again wasn't too much of a stretch even though my glass knees weren't too keen on the idea. I'm hooked again now.

CLEARER VOICE

We'll have to 'out' ourselves for our new lifestyle commitments, by telling our friends and family – and, depending on the nature of our work, our colleagues – as it may change the expectations others have of us. We may need to take the lead in this and be confident in doing so.

WHY?

- It's tough, but keeping quiet and pretending is, as we discovered, unsustainable. We'll be fearful that, if we do tell, we'll be perceived as boring even if we don't believe we are. In a work context, we may feel we're being judged negatively. I've been in this situation on several occasions, where I was expected to drink to be 'part of the team' and criticised for refusing to take part.

- Our lifestyle focus can impact our social life. Especially if those pre-menopause relationships thrived on eating red meat, boozing and blowing smoke rings. Telling all may mean the invites 'dry up' with us. For Kate and me, this happened. But we learned to adjust. We did different things. It was far from the end of the world we once imagined it would be. Rather, it turned out to be a fascinating new world.

- We have nothing to apologise for. In pursuing a more considered and healthier lifestyle we're supporting our partner to avoid health risks brought on by the menopause. We're doing what a partner should do. Not to mention benefitting our health too.

o o o

If we follow this plan, we'll be well and truly off the eggshell path.

Carving out a menopausal and post-menopausal lifestyle is a long-term endeavour, and one that needs us to commit to and pursue together. In doing so, what must work is a pattern. Not a monastic commitment to tedium, but a base from which we'll occasionally step away, knowing we'll need to step back again. All with a clear view of what we're gaining, not what we appear to be losing. As Kate stated, we need to get control first to be able to let it go occasionally. Thereafter, we'll need to support one another, each being our collective conscience as needed.

Committing to and maintaining our new lifestyle often won't be easy. But as Kate stated, it's an investment. Like all investments there's risk; but we're relying on our own resolve rather than mysterious forces. It's in our hands.

6

MOODS

During the menopause, a woman's moods can frequently change and, at times, can become more extreme. This can have a significant effect on their relationships – especially that with their partner.

MOODS: KATE

UPS AND DOWNS

Our hormonal cycle is often blamed for the ups and downs many of us experience during our first phase of womanhood. As much as we hated it, there are times during the menopause we'd take that familiar cycle back in a heartbeat. We're on an emotional rollercoaster that isn't letting us off until it's done. Our fluctuating hormones are in a state of decline and are quite literally messing with our head. Our body has got very used to them being around since puberty and really doesn't like giving them up.

Menopausal mood swings take us from tears to rage and back again in moments. These emotions are as exhausting as the remorse that often follows; that awful moment when we realise that our response to something was unreasonable, or that the annoyance or drama were out of proportion to the event that caused them.

This awareness can come moments, hours or even days later.

When we're in our extremes, the intensity can feel like we're careering down the frozen course of a skeleton bobsled; bright lights, moving quickly, loud noises (most of which emerge from us), being shaken and bumped with that sense of running on the very outer limits of control, struggling at every turn. In the slump that follows, awareness, stress, anxiety and desperation fill the void. And then begins the next emotional cycle.

IT'S NOT ME, IT'S YOU!

The start of this symptom is often cloaked in justification to our self: the kids were driving me crazy, my elderly parent was being difficult or work was stressful. Perhaps our partner was meant to do something, and they didn't do it (my memory is like a colander so I can't criticise Neil for forgetting anything, but somehow I manage it, occasionally). Within a moment the shouting begins, or we feel the deep well of tears rising. The sense of being slighted or let down is all-consuming, and their attempts at explaining the situation is only making things worse. We've escalated from a steady state to literally the end of the world in a moment.

In these circumstances, our partner can feel like the luxury of managing a straightforward pre-menstrual bad mood has passed forever, and that they're now juggling fiery, exploding coals, which can switch to sub-zero liquid nitrogen bombs at a moment's notice. Risky.

OH NO, IT'S ME!

The unpredictability of our moods is disorientating, disturbing and stressful for everyone, especially us. If we're in the rationalising phase, refusing to admit that anything unusual is occurring, we're fooling ourselves. There's a great big something going on, and facing it is the first step towards taking control.

Moods in all their extremes can impact other symptoms, aggravating them, sucking them into the swirling tornado of emotions that are part of this symptom. These include:

- Self-confidence: when we don't know what version of ourselves is going to turn up in any given moment, let alone day, we start to distrust ourselves, driving down our confidence.
- Anxiety and panic attacks: leading on from the above, when we've lost our predictable sense of self, it can cause high

levels of stress and anxiety. For some this feeling of being untethered can also cause panic attacks.

- Libido: very few of us want to strip off our kit and get sexual when we've spent the day flipping from being angry to tearful and back again. Moods also see many women go from deep insatiable desire to repulsion in the blink of an eye. It's confusing and exhausting for us, but many more times so for our partner.

Simply hoping this symptom will go away robs us of the ability to act for ourselves. It also places the bond between us and our partner under pressure. If there were hairline cracks in the relationship before the menopause began, bigger cracks and then chasms can open rapidly unless addressed.

TOXIC STRESS TANGO

One of the key issues here is that the anxiety and stress that is associated with moods and so many other menopausal symptoms are easy to dismiss, more difficult to manage and, in the long term if left unaddressed, can lead to burnout as well as a wide range of other health issues.

The symptoms we often associate with stress mirror those we can experience during menopause. They include:

- Insomnia
- Fatigue

- Loss of confidence
- Headaches
- Mood swings – yes, really!

There are a couple of reasons why stress is particularly toxic during the menopause. Firstly, stress makes symptoms worse, which in turn makes stress worse, and so it goes on.

Secondly, due to the changes in our hormones, we're less able to automatically or unthinkingly dial stress down. Instead, it's up to us to take positive action.

There are specific biological reasons for this, primarily centring around our adrenal glands. These small glands do important work – they produce both adrenaline and cortisol, our 'fight, flight or freeze' hormones. In addition to this, during the menopause they helpfully step in to support our ovaries in the production of progesterone, to keep them at the levels we've become accustomed to.

However, in moments of stress – and let's face it, menopause can be seriously stressful – our adrenal glands stop helping and simply focus on their day job, producing those hormones that will help us run fast or jump high. This is doubly problematic, because oestrogen and progesterone make a stress-countering contribution: oestrogen helps with the production of serotonin, our 'happy hormone', and progesterone, for the majority, has a calming effect on us as our 'comfort' hormone.

It's not surprising, therefore, that the impact of stress during the menopause is more extreme than it was prior to our perimenopause. We therefore must consciously remove ourselves from the situation. The choice to calm down can only be made by us.

There are several things we can do to help.

▶ KATE'S ACTION PLAN

STOP PANICKING!

The very first thing we need to do is stop panicking about what's happening and its potentially damaging impact on our relationships. Easy to say. Panicking helps no one: it makes us anxious, amplifies stress and increases cortisol. Also running around like a headless chicken, arms flapping, shouting and/ or sobbing, is never a great look.

WHY?

- It's time to be the brilliant adult we are, admit the impact of our unpredictable moods and plan what to do about them. Remorse only keeps us trapped and small.
- We might apologise, but we're not about to beg forgiveness or compromise ourselves. We didn't choose these symptoms, but we can choose what happens next.

TRIGGER, UNHAPPY

The fluctuations in our moods seem to come from nowhere, but this is not always the case. It's time to unpick our moods, to find out what's really going on, to understand if certain environments, behaviours, food or drinks trigger them. Minor irritants can also be magnified at this time, often irrespective of the situation. Bawling someone out at the first acquaintance because they slurped their cappuccino will have us scrubbed off the guest list for next time, possibly for all time.

WHY?

- Triggers can come from anywhere and anything. They're often tied to things we already find annoying, no matter how trivial. There are also the less obvious triggers such as processed foods or sugary, caffeinated drinks and alcohol. Chocolate was mine – much as I love it, it was lethal for my stability.

- Triggers aren't always obvious; we may have to look harder and deeper. What we think may have been the trigger may instead turn out to have been masking the real one.

- Once we know what our triggers are, we can systematically start to remove them or at least reduce them. If one of our triggers is our partner not replacing the toilet roll, this is relatively easily resolved. However, if it's our toddler refusing to put their shoes on in the morning or our boss micromanaging us, it's a little trickier. We need to consider what we can do to shield ourselves from the impact of these triggers.

WHAT HAPPENS NEXT?

Some moods do however seemingly come out of nowhere, or the trigger fires before we have a chance to remove or reduce them. When this occurs, we need to have a plan. Put simply, we might not be able to control the symptoms, but we can control what happens next. This will not only moderate our moods but also our stress. It's a win-win that gives us another helping of that all-important control.

WHY?

- Some environments are more stress-inducing than others. If we find ourselves in a place where we can feel things getting too much, it's time to physically take ourselves away. We can always go back when we have a handle on things, should we wish to.
- The solutions are easy to find. They include:
  - Mindfulness, meditation and breathing exercises. They're extremely effective at regulating a rush of hormones. I'd recommend everyone to regularly practice mindfulness – it helps with many other symptoms including anxiety, depression, panic attacks and insomnia.
  - Fluid. Cortisol and other spent hormones can be flushed

out by drinking lots of water. It has to be water – we mustn't be tempted by a sweet fizzy drink, coffee or caffeinated tea.
   – Sensory shocks. They can snap us out of our spiral, such as putting ice-cold water on our face or eating something incredibly sour. Our brain can only focus on one sensory experience at once and it chooses the new stimulus, thereby creating a necessary break.

TALKING... AGAIN

Talking is the pathway out of all tricky situations in a relationship. Not talking is the lead weight that keeps us anchored in a bad space. For the most part we don't talk about the impact of our moods enough, as the lack of awareness drives embarrassment for us and the fear of judgement from others. But having got here, this is where things start to change. Talking helps us manage not just the symptom and its triggers but also the impact of both, which can be corrosive. There are many ways to tackle this, and they'll beneficially develop over time. The critical thing is to start.

WHY?

• It's easier to adjust any part of the chain reaction brought on by menopausal mood swings if we fully understand it. We need to follow the earlier actions in this plan, to enable us to talk about how our moods are showing up, what our triggers are and how this is impacting our everyday life together.

- It allows us to give our partner blanket permission to step in and flag that things are getting out of hand if we find ourselves at the outer limits, sobbing or screaming. If we're feeling aggrieved and are shouting, a pre-agreed squeeze of the hand or the use of an affectionate, personal term or action can be just the intervention that's needed. Whatever it is, if we agree to act on the signal, we must take notice: shut up, step away, breathe out, bite the lemon in our drink and de-escalate. We must put the effort in to break the cycle. If we don't, we risk building mutual resentment. However, if we take the cue, it can strengthen the bond, as trust is built through our partner's preparedness to listen and support.

- The more we manage, the more we'll trust we can manage. At the extreme end of the spectrum of moods, menopausal rage is particularly unsettling, especially if we were generally calm before the menopause began. I recall once pacing around the edge of a local pub garden like a newly caged lion over a particularly minor disagreement with a friend. I was out of control and couldn't get a handle on it. After an hour of waiting for it to subside, Neil stepped in, brought me my jacket and quietly suggested I go home. This was, on reflection, the cue for me to pay to see a gynaecologist – it couldn't continue like this. I needed to take additional action.

- However desperate our moods can feel at times, we shouldn't overlook the power of humour to break or offset them. Neil has always been able to make me laugh. Not by telling jokes, but often just with simple, beautifully timed observations. Over our time together he's perfected a way of identifying humour in the extremes of my moods. He's undeterred in trying to reveal it, starting small, trying out different avenues, until he cracks it. And me. In that moment, any dark cloud evaporates, and we're off in a different direction. Like every strategy we may deploy, it's not a failsafe. Sometimes it doesn't work, sometimes it's just enough. But, when it works, it's marvellous.

o o o

All told, managing menopausal mood swings is far from easy. If we're in that space we'll know; if we haven't reached it yet, it's best to be aware that it's a common symptom. If it's present, it's vital to be able to recognise the triggers and how they appear, and to understand what can be done about them, individually and together. The support of our partner is necessary and appreciated, but with mood swings, we must – for ourselves – always be in the driving seat.

MOODS: NEIL

MOOD MAPS

A mood is something we can't be without. There's no neutral state, 'moodless'. We're going to be feeling *something*. Even when we're not feeling much at all, devoid of emotion, flat, we're in an ambivalent or unresponsive 'mood'.

There are lists of such states, adjectives that describe how we are at a point in time: happy, gloomy, reflective, pensive, playful, sad, fearful. You know the kind of thing. We'll detect and often articulate the mood of others. "You're a grumpy bugger today, Malcolm." Sorry, Malcolm, just needed an example. In addition to people, we ascribe moods to art forms such as music, painting, sculpture, film, buildings and spaces. Moods are, in short, everywhere.

The world isn't split into relatively un-moody people who have successful relationships on the one hand, and those prone to evident, oscillating moods who don't on the other. Nor do all the moody people shack up together as they understand each other, as no one else knows what they're going through. Those more prone to rapidly changing and more pronounced moods move freely among us. They may already *be* us.

Being close to someone, we get to know their emotional patterns, whether that be from time of day, media interactions, particular events or even atmospheric conditions. Or of course, as is usually the case, a combination. It helps us to safely navigate the relationship, knowing when to appear and when to be less visible. It becomes unconscious; we code it in.

When the pattern is broken, we're likely to be off balance, our prompt/response system not much use to us. We make the wrong moves and feel disoriented. While rare, we may even feel resentful: how *dare* our partner change without full and proper advance warning, in triplicate?

So, let's introduce the menopause, so we can take all the emotional certainties and patterns in our relationship, wrap them in a bedsheet and chuck them out of the window.

STORM BEFORE THE CALM

'Menopausal' doesn't describe a mood. Moods are a symptom of the menopause that can stand alone but are frequently part of a broader experience. Their origin is often within the basket of other menopausal goodies, the effects of which are understandable by us all. After several nights of disturbed sleep, for example, anyone would feel irritable and begin to develop anxiety about the need for sleep, further exacerbating the problem.

As we've moved through this book, it's hoped that an appreciation has developed that the menopause changes everything for a woman – physical, emotional and, for some, spiritual. We know from the catalogue of material published that the menopause is highly likely to alter the nature of the moods experienced by our partner, the frequency and unpredictability of their change, their severity and the triggers that drive the fluctuations. Kate's experience certainly matched this description.

That's the good news – we know menopausal moods are probably coming and what will happen. Even if we're often drawn to ask on occasions, "Bloody hell, where did *that* come from?" Only we don't know when the symptoms will appear and to what degree. Just that the old relative certainties, as far as they were, are over.

Mood swings can also result from a frustration with aspects of, or the whole, menopause experience. So rather than being a specific symptom, however integrated, they're a reaction. How would we cope with sweats or flooding in the middle of an important work presentation, entirely forgetting a vital appointment or even a whole business trip, a kilo gained since yesterday lunchtime's cheese toastie, or perhaps a desperate need for the toilet while teeing off at the 15th hole (which is furthest from any facility or privacy)? Golf – stupid game, anyway (for anyone that's seen *The Sopranos*).

While we're about to embark on an up-to-eight-year roller-coaster ride through hostile territory, unpredictability means there are likely to be periods of calm and balance too. We simply don't know when. We may even be forgiven for thinking at such times that perhaps stability has returned and that maybe the whole menopause is over.

The timing and potential severity of our partner's moods aren't simply an excuse for us to disappear. Our partner doesn't want to be like this; it's not a conscious choice, they're stuck with it. We need to understand that a ferocious mood on their part isn't a rejection of us, but a request for our help and understanding. Just perhaps not a rational or calm one.

Faced with an unpredictable landscape, there are several things we can do to help our partner's menopausal moods.

▶ NEIL'S ACTION PLAN

A BIT MORE CONVERSATION, A BIT LESS ACTION

Yes, the first and most important strategy is to talk. Kate mentioned it in her action plan, and we devoted a whole earlier chapter to the importance of it. When it comes to talking with our partner during the menopause, no subjects are off the table. It's usually a question of timing, especially so with moods. If raising the subject is like flicking a match into a bag of fireworks, we may well be forgiven for developing a protective hesitancy at times. The last thing someone struggling with understanding or controlling their mood needs to hear is that they're being unreasonably moody. It's a hugely contextual live-and-learn thing.

WHY?

- As our partner can't rationalise how they're behaving when a menopausal mood swamps them, when it's subsided we'll need to be able to explain to them what happened and the outcomes. Not to embarrass them or score points, but so they can understand what happens in such instances and are able to request support in the future that may help. This isn't judgement on our part, and we must be careful to ensure our partner knows this.

- We'll need to agree boundaries, to know under what conditions we have their permission to step in and what we'll need to do if the line we identify is crossed. There'll need to be an emergency exit we're both happy to sign up for, something we both agree to do. We'll never get to that point through telepathy.

TRIGGERS, HAPPY

We can recognise the triggers for our partner's mood changes and do what we can to ensure the triggers are not present, or if they're unavoidable, to help manage them. It requires awareness on our part, and a preparedness to act. We're not just there to point at the volcano erupting, but to find a safe path away.

WHY?

- Prevention rather than cure. We can be proactive. It's likely that we'll be able to spot triggers or patterns that our partner won't, or that they won't be in the frame of mind at the time to analyse rationally. At the right moment, we can raise them with her. In the temptation to experiment to prove a hunch, however, we should avoid creating a living laboratory in which our partner is the unsuspecting subject.

- It's possible that we'll be the accidental or responsible trigger from time to time. Which means we'll need to get used to the fact that we'll be called an "arse" on occasions. It's all about us, naturally. Because while it's not a blame environment, it'll often be our fault, regardless. We'll have to learn not to take it personally. Of course, we can't rule out that we may actually *have* been an arse on more than one occasion. Either for what we did or didn't do but should have done. Even if we were or weren't supposed to do it. To some extent we all step into that place sometimes. But we must ensure we don't become a tax-paying, passport-holding resident.

TRIGGER THYSELF

We also need to beware of, and manage, our *own* mood triggers. Which also means talking to our partner about them. Situations can sometimes degenerate quickly, each of us contributing to a negative state in the other and so on until, only one of us walking away can solve it. If this is repeated, after a while one of us will walk away for good.

WHY?

- As suggested above, we can be the cause. Our moods can be a trigger for our partner's moods. By understanding and controlling our moods we're removing a trigger for our partner.

- We're in *this* relationship where the menopause has intervened, requiring a unique response for this relationship only. Most of us by this time in our life have experienced at least one problematic relationship, whether that be a partner, a work colleague, friend or family member. One where, perhaps, we yielded too often, didn't stand our ground or allowed a situation to deteriorate before we acted. Or the opposite of each. As a result, we promised ourselves we'd handle things differently in the future. We therefore need to make sure we're not acting as though we're in a previous relationship, using the present to right the mistakes of the past.

MAKE PEACE, NOT WAR

Our key role regarding menopausal mood changes is as peacemaker. As we covered in the earlier 'Expectations' chapter, this may, if we've ever felt that at the end of a given period that the scores should always be equal, require us to discard our sense of pre-menopausal balance when it comes to right and wrong. Our peacemaking strategy may need to comprise two stages: first, the gestures Kate referred to, the signals that we use to gently indicate that our partner's mood is escalating, that we're there for them and love them, but that they need to regain personal control. The second follows in the next point.

WHY?

- Someone must. We need to develop and perfect the art of offering the hand of peace, whatever injustice we may feel about the exchange that just took place. It's not about us, of course. We're doing it for the team. Because while we may not find the patterns we once understood, we may get to recognise the signs, at least. Most importantly, we can spot and name the event and be ready to respond.

- Peacemaking shouldn't be confused with avoiding saying what we need if we feel we have a valid position, becoming habitually submissive or simply rolling over on every occasion for an easier life. All these practices can build needless resentment that will only surface later. There's a confidence in offering the hand, an assurance that a situation can be diffused with equal regard for both parties.

- It's a shortcut to normality. Kate and I agreed that, as much as there was a risk that it may provoke as well as resolve, that if I felt she was being unreasonable or overly reactive at any time, or that her emotional response was widely disproportionate, I could call it out. Kate and I therefore had a safe expression we both recognised and understood. There was often a moment of processing on Kate's part, a plateau, that then usually led to a gradual climbdown from the summit. We worked on the basis that within every mood change was a nub of stability and reason, we simply needed to access it to neutralise the rest.

• As Kate suggested, gentle humour can be a pathway to peace. It's a gift that keeps on giving.

RATIONALISE, DON'T CRITICISE

When the situation has calmed, the second stage of our peacemaking strategy is that we need to ensure the analysis happens: why did our partner's mood change, what were the triggers, the factors we couldn't control, what we may have each done differently? It's all too easy just to get on with whatever was happening just before it flared.

WHY?

• Every sudden mood change, when together, is an opportunity to gain further understanding and control that should never be passed up.

• We must learn together. It'll mean learning about and understanding both of us. As men, we'll be better for it.

• As a famous historian once remarked, those who don't remember the past are condemned to repeat it. We'll probably repeat it but will get progressively better at handling it.

EXPLAIN, DON'T COMPLAIN

We'll have a role as the 'explainer', for when our partner's volatile moods reveal themselves in the company of others. We may have got used to the new unpredictability, but others may not. If our partner has flipped over the drinks table in a fit of pique and slammed the door on the way out, we may be left facing a puzzled crowd awaiting a reason. And the only reason we can give is a calm explanation of what's happening and why. Our circumstances will be important in framing what we say. We'll need a ready-made script in our head for such occasions, hoping we'll never need it, but there and practised if we do.

WHY?

- We may be the only one in our relationship left in the room, so it'll be on us. Whether we like it or not.
- We can't expect our partner to react to a trigger, go through a mood change, and then also be the one to calmly set out what happened and why. A 'you made the mess, you clear it up' approach on our part will be a clear signal to our partner that we don't want to be in the relationship, even if we do.

MASTER OURSELVES

Finally, we can be selfless. Living with a partner with mood swings, we'll find ourselves experiencing similar emotional states through frustration or an inability to understand or deal with the emerging situation. Our own emotional state can become affected by the loss of certainty and stability. At times, we may feel that we've been unfairly penalised. We aren't lucky enough to be immune from outside influences. When feeling aggrieved, we often conveniently forget the times that our partner turned us around and dragged us out of our own self-induced, self-obsessed grunt.

WHY?

- We are, as is the theme of this book, in this together. Even if it's not made clear in brochures that the menopause is a *shared* change. It's often difficult for anyone to face up to the challenge of being required to change because of another. We never asked for it, nor do we especially feel the need to change if we were happy as we were. But we're not going back.
- Quite simply, for us as men, mastering ourselves is far easier than going through the menopause.

o o o

As we've made our way through these chapters and learned about our partner's menopausal experiences, a golden rule of menopause for men has arisen:

Whatever element or combination of elements of our partner's menopause we think is difficult for us to handle, it's never as difficult as it is for them.

Our partner's mood changes are the ultimate example of this.

We must never feel as though the odds are stacked against us, and that if we emerge in one piece it's because we're nothing short of a superstar. If we think this way, it's a long way back. If we ever make it back at all from such a place. It may be considered that the entire purpose of this book is to ensure we don't fall into such a trap of your own making. There's too much of a positive contribution for us to make to let that happen.

7

NIGHT AND DAY

During the menopause, a woman's sleep patterns may become severely disrupted, impacting their night, which in turn impacts their day, and then the following night – and so on. Their partner's sleep patterns may be similarly affected, with a possible negative impact on the relationship.

NIGHT AND DAY: KATE

ANXIOUS MOMENTS

I'm not talking about the Cole Porter track performed by Fred Astaire if you like old movies, or Lady Gaga if you like the modern version. I'm talking about the impact of menopausal symptoms that haunt you at night and then impact your days.

Before the menopause, the night was a time for socialising, raucous parties and wild sex, followed by long and restful sleep. Somehow the days and nights were separate, carefully demarcated zones in which entirely different things happened.

Once the perimenopause begins, that separation seems to blur and the days and nights bleed into one another. Continuous and inexplicable fatigue drives how we experience our days, a sense of not being in control, as though our minds are swimming through soup, while repeated interruptions from our symptoms dog our nights.

The rising anxiety of being in this space, feeling as though we're failing or spiralling out of control, is compounded by making poor food and drink choices; sugar, carbohydrates, caffeine and alcohol, consumed in a desperate attempt to get through the turmoil until the day's end. Which, when it arrives, bites us on the backside, with no let-up as we stare at the ceiling for the duration of yet another night. The cycle feels endless. The only thing that changes is that our other menopausal symptoms are dragged into a darker place. Cue anxiety, panic attacks and depression. Sleep deprivation is extremely serious, not just in itself but in what it brings.

NO MORE WINKS

One of the first signs for many that we're entering perimenopause is difficulty sleeping. In medieval times, sleep deprivation was a torture, often used on women to get them to admit being a witch. It renders us irrational, emotional and unable to think clearly. It can feel the same during the menopause, only without the witch-finder general.

As this experience is equally likely to be the result of a stressful life amongst other things, we're prone to attributing its onset to something else: a taxing project at work perhaps, or family or lifestyle issues. The very last thing we think about is the menopause. Should we have had a flicker of such a thought, it's often dismissed immediately with "no, impossible – I'm far too young". Looking back, this was me. As mentioned in the introduction, I was 42, and we had a one-year-old and a three-year-old. There was always an alternative reason, but the anxiety never left, and sleep became elusive.

I'd slept like a baby all my life until this point: I regularly fell asleep on the back seat of my parents' car before we reached the end of the street, on many poolsides on a towel while I waited for my race at endless swimming galas; I even fell asleep on ferries in high seas. Then: bam! Not anymore. Throughout my perimenopause and menopause, over a period of four years, I had four nights of solid sleep. The rest were full of snatched moments. I look back now and wonder how I functioned at all.

RED-HOT NIGHTS

Sleep-related symptoms all have a potentially negative effect on our relationship with our partner. It started with night sweats. At least, this was where my physical symptoms started for real. The undeniable sounding of the menopause klaxon, as I awoke fearing I may self-combust. The nocturnal partner to hot flushes. Both made themselves at home in my life early on in my perimenopause.

Night sweats can range from feeling a little hot, to drenching the bed. I was in the middle of this scale. They can occur once a night or multiple times. My experience was the latter. For each sweat I was woken two times, once with intense heat which caused me to throw the covers off me and onto Neil. The second was when I woke up freezing cold because I was wet from sweating, with no covers, and I'd lost considerable body heat. I would pull the covers back on, desperate for warm comfortable sleep. In the process, Neil repeatedly went from one layer of quilt to two layers and back again. Once the covers were back on, as we'd started the night, the cycle began again.

Some women who drench the bed in sweat get up, shower, change their nightwear and then change the bedding. This is extremely disruptive to both ours and our partner's sleep patterns, especially if this occurs a few times a night.

There are also the hundred rounds of the bedroom and house that comes with insomnia, as we struggle to shut down.

The constant shifting, moving and general huffing and puffing can be disruptive. Our partner may occasionally voice an objection, but listening to them contentedly snore is no comfort when we're battling with the night.

If we're experiencing those symptoms that devastate sleep patterns, they can very quickly ratchet up many of those we attribute to daytime.

All of the cognitive and emotion-based symptoms are first on the list. Our ability to be rational and think things through before responding is shredded by persistent sleep deprivation. These include but are not limited to:

- Mood swings
- Anxiety
- Depression
- Panic attacks
- Difficulty concentrating
- Memory lapses and loss of verbal recall

All these symptoms have a symbiotic relationship with our ability to sleep. Put simply, troubled days follow troubled nights.

TWO IN A BED

In managing the disruption at night from menopausal symptoms, whether occasional or chronic, it's a matter of teamwork.

We want our partner in the same bed – the spare room is where intimate relationships go to die. Which means asking them to help with our evening routine, to make sure we don't stray, and ideally have them follow it too. The mere sight of them scrolling through their phone when ours has been dark for hours will be as devastating to our attempts to shut down as us doing the same.

Teamwork needs a plan and commitments. We'll need to work on and agree the plan together and make commitments to ourselves and one another. There is, at least, a mutual benefit in it all working.

One small thing to consider when planning: if we have young children, as ours were when my menopause started, we'll need to ensure that we both share the burden of *their* night-time sleep issues. If there's an assumption that as the menopausal woman, we'll always manage the children's sleep because we're up anyway, we're embedding a behaviour that won't serve us well. We're both parents. Just like we teach the kids in the playground, we take it in turns.

Sleep issues often sit at the heart of an extreme menopause. If we can solve the sleep symptoms, many of the others will become instantly manageable. Fortunately, there are some things we can do.

▶ KATE'S ACTION PLAN

NIGHT SWEATS: DETECT AND AVOID

Dealing with night sweats – and hot flushes – means we need to become a very organised and systematic detective. We must seek out those things that disturb our hormonal patterns and cut them out. The items below are probably more 'what' than 'why' but they're all doable.

WHY?

- What we eat and drink (in terms of both content and timing) has a considerable impact on this symptom. There is no hiding from it. Big meals in the evening are out. If our body is busy digesting, it'll undoubtedly be a difficult night.
- Sugar, alcohol and caffeine are stimulants. None of these are helpful when we're trying to calm our body. At least for the first period they should be cut out completely for a couple of months. After that we can reintroduce them one at a time to see if they have any effect.
- Exercise is fantastic, as we've covered, but anything that raises our body temperature and increases adrenaline is best to be avoided for several hours before bed. If we're sweating *before* we get between the sheets, it's only going one way.
- Hot baths or showers before bed are no longer soothing: they're sweat-inducing.

- The bedroom must be kept cool, not cold, as it'll help moderate the first awakening. And those that follow.

INSOMNIA: PLAN AND COMMIT

This symptom has a long tail. We need to be thinking about winding down for bed hours before we do. Skipping the steps until ten minutes before bed is only going to end in us staring desperately at the ceiling at 2 a.m. No one needs that. The list below is also more 'what' than 'why' – but again, we can do each of them.

WHY?

- Turn. The. Tech. Off. This means our phone, tablet, laptop, watch, desktop and any other new-fangled gadget that has emerged since the time of writing. The blue light emitted by each is the death knell for our circadian rhythm. For keeping us awake, its worse than next door's impromptu 80s revival party. If you're like me, turning your phone off is more difficult than I want to admit to. Neil has on more than one occasion reminded me: "Kate, you said no phones…" Which of course I manage like a grown-up. See the chapter on 'Moods'.
- The previous point applies to our partner too. We can't be looking over their shoulder as they passively scroll. Blue light, like smoking, doesn't just impact the one doing it.
- The complexity here is not just the blue light, it's the

behaviour that follows which compounds the problem. I look at my phone under the ruse of checking tomorrow's weather. If you're British, you'll understand. I then find myself looking at messages and emails, which before I know it have kicked off a thought process. It may be an insight or inspiration, but it's more often a prompt to deal with something that just won't wait till morning. Once this starts, there's no going back, no gentle unwind. We're writing emails in our head. Sleep will be a memory from yesterday and remain elusive.

- Mindfulness can be an incredibly effective aid to sleeping if used daily as part of a programme. This doesn't mean dipping into it as and when; it means doing it every day, so that we can seamlessly activate it at night as a learned behaviour. We also need to think carefully about the irony at this time of seeking out mindfulness apps on our phone: we give, and we take away.

- To this day if Neil and I can't sleep, we reach for magnesium. We need it to help us process vitamin D, but it very handily helps us sleep as well. It can be absorbed through the skin via sprays (which we've used regularly) or taken in tablet form. Be aware, its effect is subtle; it doesn't deliver a knockout. As with any supplement, professional advice is needed before taking, along with a careful check on the dose.

- Cognitive behaviour therapy (CBT) has been proven to positively impact night sweats and hot flushes.

- The devastating impact of long-term sleep deprivation can prompt us to bring in the big guns, to visit our doctor and ask about HRT.
- If for medical reasons we can't take HRT or it's not our preferred option, there are other solutions. There are a wide range of alternative therapists that can provide support.

o o o

With open communication on which symptoms we're suffering from, their severity and their impact – together with a plan, commitment and support from our partner – we can begin to separate our expectations and experiences of nights and days once again, limiting the negative effects of one on the other. With enough sleep we can face the day, and with a degree of control during the day we can face the night. Disturbances will, with focus from us and assistance from others, become a feature we can sometimes master – and one day, quite possibly, laugh about.

NIGHT AND DAY: NEIL

FOG OFF, MENOPAUSE

The Stone Age mental wiring to which we previously referred has been honed over 300,000 years of evolution – seven million years including Homo sapiens's ancestors.

The circadian and diurnal rhythms of our biology ensure

our factory settings regulate our days and nights, adjusting our behaviour and expectations accordingly. We instinctively respond to light and dark. Which is why prolonged night shifts are so damaging to the human body, and an '*out* out' club night takes the following week to get over. At least, it does now.

As Kate has identified, menopause rudely interrupts these simple patterns. For us both.

As partner, the support we provide to our partner during menopause can't be a binary consideration, as in we're doing it or not. As considered before in this book, it needs to be subtle, flexible and responsive. We need to read the signals and to distinguish them from noise. Which is far easier said than done in the 'fog of menopause'.

It would be all the easier if we knew that the day or night were tougher than the other. Yet as with all things menopause, that would be *far* too straightforward and hence manageable.

We must consider the effect of night on day, day on night. An unbelievably poor, disturbed sleep would tee anyone up for a big day like a sedated sloth. That moment when we must get out of a bed we've only just literally settled into after torrid insomnia. A little like our first daughter, who, when just a year or two old, would scream a short-haul flight near-out of the sky and then magically slip into a blissful snooze as the wheels hit the runway.

Similarly, an irritable day of misunderstanding and overreaction, missed meetings and overlooked must-dos, inexplicable sweats and moments of overwhelming brain-fog don't exactly set our partner on course for a gradual slide into a baby-like sleep.

Very often, such days drive a desire for consumption of the last things our rational brain would opt for, as we covered in the 'Lifestyle' chapter: caffeine, sugar, alcohol or worse, or all the above.

NIGHT DIVIDES THE DAY

We may be forgiven for starting with the day: surely that must be the toughest time? It's twice as long as the night, to begin with. Especially as we've now grown out of Northern Soul all-nighters. And we're probably somewhere else for much of it, not there to lend assistance beyond phone support (work-dependent) for our partner, even if we wanted to.

Yet for us all, the day provides many hiding places, some in the plainest of sight. We can lose ourselves amid crowds and situations, moving stealthily between them and dipping out as we need. While our partner may be required to be somewhere with work or pinned to the desk in front of a camera and screen in a barrage of appointments, there are often spaces in between. There may even be the opportunity to turn the camera off to allow a scream, silent or otherwise.

Yet unless we're both working at home, there'll likely be a significant separation between us during the day. Our partner will need to manage their way through it themself, slaloming through colleagues unable or unwilling to talk about or even recognise the menopause (which is almost all of them), navigating a workplace unsympathetic to anyone but the mythical 'average person' – therefore meaning no one – and perhaps a corporate culture still trying to get its head around the before-and-after of pregnancy, let alone anything beyond.

There are exceptions in each regard, of course.

So, despite the nooks and crannies of respite the day offers, it's not necessarily easier than the night. It's not our 'time off' the menopause, either. We may be reduced to remote support, but it's vital support, nonetheless.

DAY DIVIDES THE NIGHT

So, the night must be easier then? Not necessarily. It's damned difficult for our partner falling asleep on the sofa in front of a suitably tame television programme and then, as soon as their head hits the pillow, feeling awake enough to thread a thousand needles, listening to us snuffle and grunt into the claustrophobia of the smallest hours. We deny snoring, naturally. Who doesn't?

The consciousness of needing to be unconscious to ensure we can get through tomorrow just makes it all the harder to switch off. Sleep remains a mystery to us, as something we've no awareness of enjoying until it's over. Yet all the while craving it intensely.

At night – through the audible expression of frustration,

the sudden flinging back of the quilt during a raging sweat, repeated visits to the toilet in the hope that an entirely empty bladder might do the trick, the reading light and casual turning of pages – our partner has only one person to be annoyed at. They feel somehow betrayed that *they're* the tired one and yet *we're* the one asleep. Unlike the day, there are no corners in which to hide or escape chutes into the anonymity of a crowded street. They're empty too, save for other insomniacs.

Whether it's insomnia pure and simple or a combination of symptoms, the menopause will eat greedily into our partner's night. And, by association, ours.

Sometimes we're not dealing just with the 'tossing and turning' (in this context, I'm never sure of the difference), but it could drive the need to change the bedclothes entirely. We're talking potentially flu-like sweat levels, soaking sheets that not even fresh clothes and a towel can resolve. That's a whole new level of disturbance we haven't experienced since pre-teen years when we dreamed of peeing in a field to find it wasn't actually a field. In which instances we stood by and watched our parents do the sheet-changing, their frosty glares tinged with a distant memory of themselves doing the same.

TO EVERYTHING, A SEASON

That's the Monday to Sunday. We shouldn't forget, either, that the seasons have an impact, in which the length of the days vary, along with temperature and humidity. Weight gain and uncontrollable sweats don't sit easy with a summer dress on a balmy evening where everyone's halfway through their second bottle of rosé. Each. Quiltless and airless nights merely make insomnia worse.

Managing the situation over a long period, in which the effects can be cumulative and create symptoms for us both, doesn't mean heading for the spare room. That degree of rejection only compounds the problem. In particular, as the bed is not only a place of rest, but the intimate space, away from the distractions of daily life – however thin the walls.

That prompts us to offer another golden rule of menopause for men: absolutely nothing we do can ever appear, in even the slightest form, to look or feel to our partner like punishment.

The sense of injustice will linger long and dangerously; it'll always resurface. Let he who has not been a pillock at night at some point cast the first stone. Put it down, you're kidding yourself.

To be clear, our partner hasn't suddenly become a dependent child. They are, and will remain, an intellectually capable, rational adult who needs a little additional help with factors sometimes beyond day-to-day and night-to-night control.

There are three key things we can do to support our partner through the differing impacts of the menopause during daylight and night hours.

🎬 NEIL'S ACTION PLAN

VERSATILITY

We must be ready for rapid adaptation through day and night. Our response isn't about being consistent. It means fighting the fact that we're brought up on linear problem-solving methods: definition, plan, delivery and review (anyone who has done Six Sigma will come out in hives at this point). It's all those years at work, particularly for those who've laboured in a corporate environment, driving out uncertainty until we have something left that's uninteresting but manageable. Scrap all that – it's not going to work here. The ball's being thrown against mattress springs and we're going to have to catch it.

WHY?

- It's not about theories and ideas for us. We need to be able to react quickly and instinctively. Even if on occasions we get it wrong, the speed and willingness of our response, even where it's a small gesture or exchange, will be a mark of our commitment to help and support.
- If the menopause is unique for every woman, constantly evolving, so too must be a man's response. We're simply mirroring the experience with our response.

PRACTICALITY

In being ready, we must then be practical to a fault. Which means doing things we can do, that are entirely possible. We don't even need to refer to the menopause – we're just being a good partner. We should start with what we know we can do and work outwards from there. Small achievements, visible signs of progress; they're all-important indicators of interest and support.

WHY?

- It's all achievable. During the day we can make sure there's a rest space available, appreciated (and healthy) food and drink within reach, a second phone to act as a 'menopause hotline' if needed for when we're not present, a daily jointly prepared end-of-day list of what must happen tomorrow, a range of measures agreed and understood for when their mood flares or a reaction appears entirely irrational. At night, it can mean having a process for when sheets need changing at 3 a.m.: clean sheets and nightwear on hand, waiting space for partner while bedding changed, double sheets to avoid need to change quilt cover, low-level lighting to aid sleep when it's all sorted.
- We're vulnerable too. Revealing that to our partner can break down barriers and prompt conversation. We may sometimes goof it up, even if we only occasionally admit it

to ourselves, but these situations are never a prompt to brag about being useless. We're far from that and we know it.

EXTENSIVITY

We must provide support through a range of channels for when we're present and when we're not. Because just as our partner's menopause doesn't acknowledge days and nights, it doesn't recognise our diary.

WHY?

- We're not going to be coat-tailing our partner everywhere in case something blows up – or floods. We must learn how to help while potentially being in a room full of work colleagues, being asked if we'd like another latte before our workshop continues.
- In offering extensive support to our partner, we'll be learning to manage our own frustration. Which makes us a better person and a better partner. We'll be asked for help when we're doing something, or we've just given it, or we're just tired of giving it. Particularly if, before we left the house in the morning, we'd just put the third set of sheets in the tumble dryer and missed the 06.47 train. We need to remember there's another at 07.12. And we'll get to see the sunrise.

o o o

Night and day both bring their opportunities and risks. Over the span of the menopause, while there may be fluctuations, we need to remember that the menopause is an 'always on' experience. For many years. It's quite possible we've reached this stage of the book and are still getting our heads around that. But being an amazing partner is an 'always on' experience too.

8

INTIMACY

Menopausal symptoms can play havoc with intimacy in a relationship, compounded by the difficulty we often find in talking about it or acting when it's not as we want it to be.

INTIMACY (SEX): KATE

OK, so this is the chapter everyone flicked to first. If you've started here, don't worry, you won't be the only one. As we'll explore, though, we love talking about the intimacy of others, but less so ourselves.

One of the key points we need to be aware of is that, for women, sex is about more than the act itself. It's a complex mix of emotions and experiences that lead up to and follow on from it, as well as the sex in between. It means we can't spend all day annoyed with our partner or our self and then expect fabulous, joyous sex once the opportunity arises.

This is why this chapter is called 'Intimacy' and not 'Shagging'. We left the latter behind when things got a bit (or a lot) more serious.

GOING, GOING...

Growing up, most of us never thought that our libido – sex drive – would ever be affected by anything at all. Sex seemed like a pleasure we were the first to discover. It was something many of us paid a lot of attention to, learning what we liked and didn't, what worked and didn't – for both us and them. We enjoyed the rampant freedom of our younger years when we barely got in the door before our clothes magically fell off. Roll forward a few years and things may well have changed, at least a little.

If we've been with our partner for many years, there's a chance that predictability is now a feature. They do this to us, we do that to them, then we do something together. Routine, necessity, work, exhaustion, an ever-expanding household; there'll be any number of metaphorical buttoned-up, frilly-collared, full-length, cotton floral conveniences and comforts slowly whittling away our passion. Many we'll have been increasingly responsible for, rather than them arriving by accident.

If we have kids, life and intimacy will have changed

dramatically. The opportunity for sex will have diminished. Whether that's because the kids or the babysitter are present when we tiptoe through the door, wanting to hold it together until we've at least paid and thanked the babysitter; or because our kids don't ever seem to have understood the need for privacy as they unpredictably (predictably) burst through the bedroom door to tell us the time at the most inconvenient moment.

Life in general can take its toll on intimacy. The pressures of work, deadlines, the need to be permanently 'on' at the end of our tech, ready to respond to the latest issue in the actual or virtual workplace. Add to this financial worries and general exhaustion, and we can find ourselves in a place where even functional sex can be a daydream that rarely materialises for us.

A COMPLEX WEB

It's important to recognise that while our sex drive can lessen as our hormones decline during menopause, desire and the drivers behind it are far more complex.

The web of symptoms that women experience can significantly impact intimacy. Many symptoms link together to affect our sense of self and whether we think we're sexy and, for some, whether we think our partner is sexy.

I frequently speak to menopausal women who have stopped having sex with their partners because they don't themselves feel desirable.

How we feel about ourselves influences much in the bedroom, and anywhere else for that matter. Symptoms that remove the pleasure of intimacy must be addressed, not just by the woman but with their partner too. This may seem too much like hard work at the time, but the long-term benefits are considerable. Not least that withdrawal from intimacy – on either part – will only take the relationship in one direction. And it's not a good one.

The key symptoms affecting intimacy can be:

• Sleep deprivation, whether that be through insomnia or night sweats, makes us exhausted and potentially anxious. It also triggers our drive to consume carbs, fat and sugar, simply to keep us going through the long hours of the day. This in turn causes us to put on weight, which we're more prone to do at this time in life anyway.

• Hot flushes. If this is one of our symptoms then they're likely to make themselves known at the beginning of, during and after sex. Pretty much every time. They make women feel self-conscious, slippery, and drippier than a broken tap repair shop. It can be extremely challenging to be intimate while sweating excessively.

• If we have recurrent urinary tract infections (UTIs), increased susceptibility to thrush and bacterial vaginosis (BV) or incontinence, none of these make us feel sexy or in any way desirable. Medical support will be needed here and a good place to start is localised oestrogen.

- The elephant in the room: vaginal dryness, or vaginal atrophy as it's now known. It constantly amazes me that the medical profession has chosen to change the referred name of this, from something that sounds unpleasant enough to something truly terrifying. It's no surprise that women don't want to talk about it. Unless that was the intent? Vaginal dryness is incredibly common. A member of my extended family is a doctor – she says that she has at least one woman a day asking for help with this issue. For most experiencing it, it makes intercourse anywhere from sore to excruciating, tearing the delicate tissue of the vagina. The natural lubrication experienced during foreplay and throughout sex no longer happens to the degree that it did previously or at all for some women.

- Finally, many symptoms don't on the face of it directly affect our libido, but the impact of them does. If we oscillate between emotional extremes, it can be difficult to find a calm place where we can focus on this part of our lives. Equally if we have any of the brain-fog symptoms that affect our sense of who we are, this can make us feel anxious and stressed, which is never a good precursor to slipping between the sheets.

Fortunately, there's a lot we can do. As we're getting intimate together, there's a lot our partner can do too, which Neil will cover.

▶ KATE'S ACTION PLAN

LET'S TALK ABOUT SEX...

Discussing sex – talking *and* listening – can feel difficult for many of us. But when things are not going as we would want them to or that one of us seems uninterested, we owe it to ourselves and our relationship to talk about it. This means thinking through what the issue is and what the drivers might be. Importantly, too, thinking about what the solutions might be and how they might be put into action. It's a private conversation so definitely not one for a video call on the 63 bus on the way home from work or speakerphone in the office. It's also not a subject for the bedroom. This may sound counter-intuitive, but the place where intimacy is most likely to happen needs to remain free of analysis.

WHY?

- Talking about sex can lead to more and better sex, particularly during the menopause but at other times, too. Most of us would like to be able to talk about sex more often but struggle to. The fear of asking for what we want is often because we don't want to upset our partners. Menopausal symptoms add another layer of complexity. Male and female egos alike are often very sensitive when it comes to sexual antics. We all want to think that we're accomplished in this department. The law of statistics says we can't all be, but we can all, with focus and attention, be better. If we're actively talking and listening elsewhere in our relationship, we're already laying the path in extending this to intimacy.

- It can build confidence. Talking about what we do like (or did like if it's been a while) is always a great place to start. Not only will it sweeten the conversation, but it also creates a positive foundation to start from together.

- It's also about listening, as covered in the chapter on 'Talking'. Listening is insight. It can make us more caring, sensitive, adventurous – things that can make intimacy more rewarding for us both.

- It is, of course, about saying what we might like more or less of, and absolutely *not* about offering our views or opinions on the performance of our partner. Or even ourselves. It's about mutual pleasure, so it's very much an 'us' activity. No one's drive for intimacy is fired by criticism. Shouting about the issue with all guns blazing isn't going to go well either.

- Not talking about it isn't neutral, it doesn't mean it simply stays as it is. It's likely to have a negative impact. Where there may already be issues, ignoring them and hoping they'll magically disappear won't end well.

LINKS AND WINKS

We can identify what the links and micro-gestures are between us and our partner and do more of them. These are the things that tell each of us that we're valued, loved and special. They're often the small things that have become ingrained in our day-to-day: talking, empathy and gestures of love, however small, such as holding hands or a cheeky wink. They're unique to every couple and are critical to intimacy.

WHY?

- Menopausal symptoms can cause us and our partner to withdraw, breaking those links. Their absence is often felt deeply. When relationships come under strain, especially during the menopause, these gestures create a much-needed glue, maintaining our unique pattern of links that lead us along our unique pathway towards intimacy. In my darkest times, I needed these markers more than ever; they were (and remain) signals of intimacy, connectedness and understanding. I became acutely aware of both their presence and their absence. If one was missed, I became anxious, which in turn impacted so many of my other symptoms.
- Intimacy is not an isolated activity. All the links and micro-gestures draw us towards the idea and then the act of sex. They help us feel adored and wanted, not used and functional.

START OVER

Routine is a cold shower for passion. A 'starting again' mentality helps to break the familiarity and routine that may have crept in. Here's a golden opportunity to try something new, or at least return to things not done for years. It may take a little planning to carve out privacy (from family, perhaps) and time (from life), to create an environment where there's no excuse to persist with established patterns.

WHY?

- It gives both partners the opportunity to reconnect at that level; to reignite desire, whatever changes are taking place, or menopausal symptoms are raging.
- If either partner sees it as an inconvenience, it shows a lack of consideration for the other's needs. If this persists, there's a bigger conversation to be had about the future of the relationship.
- This might not be the most comfortable place to discuss this, if there's such a place at all, but if a relationship failed at some point and both partners found themselves single again, they'd both need to start again with someone new anyway. So, there's really very little to lose and a lot to gain from trying it *within* the relationship. It's a devastating logic that seems to constantly escape attention.

MAKE TIME

During menopause, time for foreplay is required more than at any point before, to quite literally get us in the mood. It's not just about the physical response, its role in building anticipation and connecting the two of us is well known. But it can often be hastened or skipped altogether. It might start with kissing, which is fantastic, but that's not the end of it.

WHY?

- Everything that's good in our lives takes time. It's absolutely no different with intimacy.
- This area in life takes some investment to keep it working. For many, it's a place where the learning, too, starts over.
- We can either see this as exciting or a chore. This is a point of choice, one of many during the menopause. We can choose to welcome the adventure, or sulk in the corner.

LUBE ON UP

If vaginal dryness is occurring, it needs to be resolved. It can't be ignored. It's extremely unlikely that it'll resolve itself without some form of intervention. Within our relationship we need to see the final steps towards sex, foreplay and lubrication as integral parts of our experience together. I don't mean commercial products in a phallus-shaped bottle, as they're full of chemicals that will upset our natural pH and cause even more discomfort. We should seek out organic and natural lubricants and moisturisers from specialist providers. They'll quite literally help everything feel like it used to. It does mean we have to get used to its application being a shared act, part of sex, not a passion-killing pause while something vaguely medical happens. They're relatively easy steps, but we must do them or this symptom can impact not just intercourse but also how we view our sexuality and our relationship as a whole.

WHY?

- Vaginal dryness makes intercourse sore and for some excruciatingly painful. Nobody wants to be in this situation.
- A loss of lubrication in this instance is not a failure to do something right. It's important that any thoughts along this line are dealt with quickly. That's about talking, again. If left to fester they can permanently damage our or our partner's willingness to try.
- Introducing an external element to sex can make it feel functional or disjointed. But the pleasure of a natural female-focused lubricant can be pivotal.
- If lubricants don't work sufficiently, it's easily treated with localised oestrogen. However, for some women this simply isn't enough, and it'll need to be part of a broader hormone treatment package. While we could go straight for the

oestrogen option, the opportunity for incremental pleasure and connection shouldn't be missed.

- If medical help is needed in the form of internal oestrogen and/or HRT we need to talk to our doctor – it's a common request and nothing to be embarrassed about.

REV ON UP

With testosterone, that is. Women have this hormone too, it's not a male preserve. If we find that our sex drive has fallen through the floor, we may need to talk to a specialist gynaecologist or Doctor able to prescribe testosterone.

WHY?

- Should we choose to take it, it's in a very low dosage. It'll lift our sex drive.
- It's important to note, however, that it's not a silver bullet. If we're having unsatisfying or disinterested sex, it won't resolve or change it. Great sex requires both partners to focus on changing, improving and keeping it interesting.

o o o

All of which means that intimacy, or at least the impact of menopause upon it, more than any other matter in this book, feels like a daunting hurdle – whether that's because of our symptoms, latent issues in our relationship or the bias and judgements associated with the menopause.

I'd be lying if I said that we sailed through it without a thought; we didn't. It was no different for us. But we focused on what we wanted and were prepared to learn together. The best advice we received: start with the easy stuff and gradually work into the more challenging areas from there. Throughout, we've always tried to keep it light when we can and save the intensity for later. Or earlier if we get the chance.

SEX (INTIMACY): NEIL

WALKING THE ANGEL-HAIR TIGHTROPE

One of the key points we need to be aware of is that, for men, sex tends to be about the act itself. It's not a complex mix of emotions and experiences that lead up to and follow on from it, it's essentially the sex in between. It means we can spend all day annoyed with our partner or our self and then expect fabulous, joyous sex once the opportunity arises.

This is why this chapter might be called 'Shagging' and not 'Intimacy'. We retained our interest in the former when things got a bit (or a lot) more serious.

As men, however, we're not accustomed to conversing about intimacy unless we're *really* accustomed to it. We may talk about it with close friends, at best. Even then, it's often not entirely comfortable. Those friends probably know our partner. If our friends, newly enlightened, look at our partner askance on the next occasion, thinking to themselves, "Wow, you like doing *that?* Who knew?", we may have overstepped a confidential boundary or two.

The 'problem page' and 'agony aunt' (interestingly, rarely uncle) have generated good business from this conundrum for decades. They've shielded many a concerned partner in a relationship, needing to explore something highly sensitive without revealing themselves. 'Asking for a friend.'

For both partners, talking about intimacy treads a delicate path between a constructive, relationship-building exchange and devastating criticism. Where it lands on the scale is usually a matter of how we hear and interpret it.

As men and women alike, we tend to believe that we're able to know what our partner wants and be able to make it happen. Anything that suggests otherwise, particularly when it comes out of the blue, can be jarring.

Even within an established relationship, talking about intimate matters is often avoided. There's a reliance on other processes for discovery – prompts, responses, reactions, body language – from which conclusions are drawn. Sometimes the wrong ones. And as we covered earlier, where there's silence, we'll make up the missing part of the story.

SLIPPERY SLOPES

The menopause, however, changes intimacy beyond the point at which talking about it is avoidable. At least, that is, without damaging consequences. When younger, and before the internet provided one-click visual access to every known (and possibly unknown) fantasy, we'd dream about the hottest, steamiest and sweatiest sex. Then, many years later, along came our partner's menopause and the wish was granted. Just not quite as we'd envisaged it.

Our partner wants to feel desired by us, just as we want them to desire us. There was a time in most relationships, usually at the outset, when both were never in question; when the pursuit of intimacy drowned out all other concerns. Even the involuntary, like eating and breathing.

Yet the menopause affects both our partner's attitude to intimacy and their physical response. As Kate has covered, symptoms include the usual suspects such as hot flushes and night sweats, insomnia, changes in body shape and anxiety. But they also introduce symptoms far less often discussed in a relationship, such as vaginal dryness, that render engaging in intimacy uncomfortable and even painful for our partner.

We must assume that in arriving at this chapter of the book, there remains a sexual dimension to the relationship, even if it has settled somewhat from those heady, perfumed days. Yet in the uncertain environment that the menopause creates, our partner may detect small signs that with the changes it brings about that we no longer feel as we once did, just as simultaneously we detect the same on their part. They prompt each other. We're not sure who started it. Yet we must always remember that our partner's emotions and responses are usually driven by biological circumstances beyond their control. The only one deflating our masculinity, therefore, is ourselves.

PONDERLUST

There are five key considerations here for how we approach talking about intimacy with our partner.

- Where we're at in our relationship. If it's a mature relationship, either in years or the way we both approach it, we may stand a greater chance of directly addressing the issues and deciding on a course of action and responding, than if it's still in the first exploratory flush when menopause hit, or even began after the menopause itself started. That said, it's quite possible that the relationship has survived for so long by consciously *avoiding* confronting anything of significance, an art seemingly mastered by our parents' generation and those before them.
- The expectations we have of one another. This may be driven by pre-relationship experience as much as by that of our present. We'll have learned from our own mistakes up to this point (yes, we made them), resolved to do things differently, promised ourselves that situations wouldn't

repeat themselves. Many of those 'notes to self' will relate to intimate matters. The hope is that a key expectation will be openness, on both our parts.

- The frequency of intimacy at the point the menopause intervenes. Our mind may flit to a weekly magazine survey asking how many times a week/month/year we have sex. In a reverse response to being asked how much beer we drink, we're minded to select a good week/month/year for our answer just as we select the week we had flu to state how many units of alcohol we consume. There'll be the frequency we *have* sex and the frequency we'd *like* to have sex. The hope is they'll be the around the same. Yet the arrival of menopause may disrupt the pattern significantly.

- The nature and quality of our intimacy. The word 'great' is often used prior to 'sex' when we're talking of it. Which is, of course, entirely subjective. It's an emotionless non-committal catch-all that rolls off the tongue without thought, protecting the other's ego. What's 'great' for one isn't always great for the other, which is at its most problematic when the two people concerned are in a relationship. Our perspective of 'great' will also change over time. Appraising one another and the outcome – which are different – doesn't have a natural time slot, the least helpful option being just after it's finished. It's a tricky subject. Now throw in the menopause, and it gets a whole lot trickier.

- Intimacy's dependent factors. They include work, children and our domestic living situation, and all the practicalities, demands and stress-related aspects of each. It was Kate's late elder brother who would say that having two young sons was the most effective contraceptive he'd known. The factors create both practical and emotional barriers to free-flowing and uninhibited intimacy. Where the window of opportunity narrows, the pressure to make it count intensifies. If this is further hampered by the intervention of the menopause, our enthusiasm or preparedness for intimacy risks shrinking and disappearing like the dot on a black-and-white television. If you remember that.

Our response to all the considerations faced will be vitally important. Whether it's direct action (changing our lifestyle, as we have covered, for example) or taking the initiative, or our attitude, in terms of listening, understanding and supporting – we must be *doing* something different and *seen* to be doing something different. That's both of us. If our partner is gaining weight and feeling anxious about it, sensing a loss of desire on our part, or bursting into a raging sweat when we apply a gentle hand, what are *we* going to do differently?

Unusually in this chapter, we'll look at things we should do and things we shouldn't. First, the things we should do.

▶ NEIL'S ACTION PLAN

UNPEEL OUR INHIBITIONS

Just as during the menopause we're having to get used to talking more, we're also having to get used to talking honestly about things we may never have broached before, other than in passing. We can start easily and simply in this area and develop the depth and range as we go. We're therefore unpeeling our inhibitions rather than shedding them, one layer at a time. It's at this time we may discover inhibitions we didn't know we had. If we don't get a response from our partner, this isn't a reason to give up. It's highly likely they're unpeeling theirs too.

WHY?

- We have to see it not as something to get away without doing, but as something that, if we don't do, our relationship won't get away with. It's up to us to initiate, develop and sustain the conversation until it is natural, even expected.
- A little like intimacy itself, therefore, the more we talk openly about it with our partner, the better we're likely to get at it and the less we have to fear. It can feel incredibly liberating – almost as though we're doing something forbidden.
- If we can talk about intimacy with our partner, we can pretty much be able to talk about anything. It's doubtful

there's a more difficult subject. It'll be a barometer of how far we've come as a couple.

CREATE A CUNNING PLAN

A degree of planning is necessary. Intentionally carving out time and opportunity are a practical necessity during the menopause, given that there are so many possible interventions from symptoms and life in general. We often use a lack of time or the obstacles of a typical day to excuse a lack of investment in intimacy. This is a slippery slope. Time will be an essential ingredient, or our plan will just intensify the stress associated, removing any last traces of romance. Importantly, it means time before, during and afterwards.

WHY?

- It can help with the removal of emotional and physical inhibitors, and the re-establishment of at least a small semblance of the consequence-free irresponsibility that will likely have characterised the early stage of the relationship. To clarify, it doesn't mean a carefully timed three minutes with two minutes either side for prep and mop-up.
- Planning is not the failure or defeat that some consider it to be. If a fabled 'dirty weekend' was intended, the hotel and travel would need to be booked, bags packed, the dog-sitter arranged. Planning and intimacy have always been closely related.

COMPLIMENT, IN EVERY SEASON

Our partner may be dealing with reduced self-esteem. There's a simple response on our part, to compliment. This can be verbal and non-verbal.

WHY?

- It's easy and effective. It's a wonder more of it doesn't happen outside of the menopause. Not paying compliments is an easy habit to get into, and a simple one to break. It's field research we can do and monitor in real time.
- It's even more helpful in the company of others.
- It's likely our partner pays us complements, and we consciously benefit.
- Credible research tells us that flattery has no limits: it's a gift that keeps on giving. Interestingly, even when we may be overdoing it and the person being complimented is aware we are overdoing it too.

GET HELP

We must develop a healthy familiarisation with some of the aids that may be required. Outside of car maintenance, heterosexual men can be incredibly uncomfortable with even the idea of lubricant, seeing it as a signal of failure in gel form. They may feel they've failed to excite (or even interest) their partner – it's all about us, again.

WHY?

- It's a simple biological fact that no matter how ready either party may be, if there's no natural assistance available an artificial nudge may be required. If it's given time to be seen as part of foreplay rather than an add-on, it'll be natural and unquestioned. If we think about it rationally, there are a heck of a lot worse things to be upset or distracted about.

- Linked to the first point of our action plan, talking about these aids is essential. Having to suddenly discuss reaching for and applying an organic lubricant to one or both of us at the pivotal moment, where any distractions can be erotically terminal, may be one of the more difficult opening gambits. But one we'll have to get over and get used to, both of which are entirely possible.

- When considering aids, we need to reference erectile dysfunction here too. In which case, on this occasion, it *is* about us. It has the potential to be made more complicated by the change in patterns of sexual desire and activity brought on by our partner's menopause. Which leaves both partners struggling to understand how to rebuild the sexual health of the relationship. In which case, for the man, the help of a doctor should be sought in addition to any of the suggestions made in this chapter.

There are also some things that *don't* constitute a helpful response.

DON'T STOP

A deferment, putting intimacy itself on pause, with a reassurance that 'we'll fancy them again when it's all over', is not an option.

WHY?

- No intimacy for around eight years? Our partner won't wait for us. And why on earth should they? a shared choice, not just ours to make.
- The menopause isn't an instant transformation for our partner. Nor is its end an instant reversion to a premenopausal state. There are no defined 'on' and 'off' points where decisions can be made. So consciously and intentionally pausing and restarting intimacy are near-impossibilities, and to think otherwise is fooling ourselves. And our partner.
- What our partner is experiencing is, with conscious choice and our involvement and support, an entirely manageable phase in their life. Together, we can work to create the moods and atmospheres to continue our intimacy, rather than putting it on hold.

DON'T GO

Leaving the relationship on account of the menopause isn't a strategy either.

WHY?

- The menopause reveals much about relationships, especially the cracks we once chose not to see. Our intimate life will yield the most telling and pronounced expression of such. If we can't handle several physical and psychological shifts on the part of our partner, we were probably already in the early stage of doubt.

- If the relationship had been tanking for many years and the menopause was the final straw, then, really, why did the self-deceit last for so long? It would be rather shameful if the menopause created the pretext for a split, conveniently offloading the responsibility on the partner – years of unmitigated idiocy on our part, finally given a pretext by her night sweats. If this was us, even in our most ridiculously self-centred moments, we'd always know that we unjustly exploited a situation to create an outcome we should have faced many years before.

- Even doubt about the future of our relationship doesn't mean it can't be faced, understood and addressed. If it takes the menopause to reveal it, then it may be something to be thankful for in both the short and longer term.

- The inclination to up sticks, should it be present, will in such instances be telling us something about ourselves. Far from a badge of courage awarded for taking the bold decision, it may hide a deeper fear of female disinterest or rejection. But we can't keep running all our lives; sooner or later we must face up to who we are and be honest with ourselves. Or being honest with our partner is never likely to happen.

DON'T FADE AWAY

The final response to reject, assuming there are no health considerations necessitating it, is one in which we might both be complicit – to let intimacy dwindle until it's too distant a memory to recall. In effect, an unintentional pause, whereby having faced much before, and still having a deep bond of trust, we lose the unique connection that intimacy brings to our relationship.

WHY?

- It's unlikely we're giving up intimacy for good. Sooner or later, there'll be a physical attraction elsewhere and our unwavering commitment to our relationship may be called into question.
- We can make the menopause part of who we are as a couple. When the menopause begins, neither of us know how long 'temporary' may mean in this regard, and as such we create a reality able to last as long as it needs. The menopause is simply a change that will, at some future point, change again. Yet without our being there for our partner, it may well be unmanageable and permanent.

o o o

Sex isn't a silent pursuit. If we're talking openly and honestly, listening, planning and taking the time we need, and developing a comfort with aids that will help us through this phase, we'll have every chance of staying intimate throughout and beyond. We may even discover things we hadn't experienced before or close off avenues that weren't working for us. It could very well be the birth of a deeper, more rewarding intimacy than we've ever known.

9

SECOND PHASE

The passing of the menopause signals the start of the second phase of womanhood. It's a time of incredible opportunity and promise, but one that requires a further evolution of the relationship.

SECOND PHASE: KATE

EYES FRONT

By the time you've got to this chapter, many of you may be feeling that this sounds like *too much hard work*. I'd be lying if I said that it wasn't hard work, especially if you're having a tough time with the menopause. But unfortunately, once it's begun there's no getting off until the ride is over, no matter how many dead drops or loop-the-loops. Which is tricky if, like me, you find rollercoasters challenging. The nausea kicks in just thinking about them.

While all the symptoms are causing havoc at the surface, there's a groundswell of change beneath. It's like an iceberg. As we've said (more than once!), if there's a hope that when it's over everything goes back to 'normal' – to the way it used to be before the menopause – it won't. It biologically can't. During the menopause, we are, and will have been for some time, becoming fundamentally different. Whether that brings on major life changes is up to us. But suffice to say, as our hormones return to their prepubescent levels, we'll begin to focus on what's important to us, what we want to do, who we want to be doing it with and where we want to be.

At the beginning of my menopause, I was terrified that it would mean the end of my marriage, that somehow the two were linked.

In hindsight, I'd some grounds for thinking this. My mum's menopause in all probability had something to do with her rejecting her relationship with my dad – of course it was never discussed. This was difficult for all of us. The more I learned about the menopause and rationalised what had happened, the more it stoked my fears.

That perceived link isn't a fact for all couples. If it was, we'd all have a break clause written into our relationships (and even marriage contracts) that meant we all became single again at this time. "Till death or menopause do us part."

It's nonsense, but it spurred me on to find a different way of being. Reflecting on it, though, a break clause for women only at this stage may be justifiable, for all the crap they'll have been through. Yes, we're keeping a tally.

HORMONE TANGO FANDANGO

Our hormones drive our monthly menstrual cycle, keep our body supple and our bones strong. They also help to give us qualities we identify as female: relationship-building, empathy and caring, in particular. Most of us are aware at even a basic level that our hormones contribute emotionally as well as physically.

It makes sense at an evolutionary level that we employ these skills to ensure both us and our offspring survive. For hundreds of thousands of years, we'd have needed to bond with others to help protect ourselves and our baby, at a time when we were incredibly physically vulnerable.

There was, and still is, during our reproductive years, a need to prioritise the safety and wellbeing of our children over ourselves. Mothers across the world do this every day, as they've always done. This may sound ridiculous if you're one of the many women who've not had children, but the response is part of being human. We'll care for others around us whether we choose that to be people or pets, regardless.

TANGO FOR ONE

Which brings us neatly to today.

As our hormones are doing the tango on the way out, these drivers lessen. In particular, our need to put others first stops being as important as it once was. What *we* want becomes paramount. We effectively elbow our way to the front of the queue where we remain for the rest of our lives.

To be clear, we don't stop caring about those around us, our priorities simply adjust. A common indicator that something has changed for women is hearing them say: "I can't be bothered with that anymore" or "it's just not that important now".

TWO CAN TANGO

As the menopause recedes, we're arriving at a junction where *we get to choose* what happens next. If we look one way and it's more tainted than a nicotine-stained bar from the 1970s, then look the other and it offers the glowing promise of something exciting, most of us would choose the latter. But focusing on ourselves takes a bit of practice, especially after all this time. We may surprise ourselves. It's been a few decades since we did. Focusing on our relationship is no different.

If we've descended into a 'rut' of same-old, same-old – or taking one another for granted without trying – we'll start to experience some issues. It's possible they'd have arisen without the menopause, but the impact of our experience will exacerbate them significantly. For many however, there'll be times when our partner tried and failed to support us, and others when they excelled. Only we can decide where the balance of effort and success lies.

While this too may seem scary, this phase in life is an opportunity that only women get. With every end, there is the possibility of new beginnings, including whether our future adventures are with or without our partner. This promise of future fun is the brilliant light at the end of the tunnel that draws us through the dark times. Like a siren it calls to us as we struggle with the storm of symptoms. We simply have to be prepared to look up and see it.

🎬 KATE'S ACTION PLAN

DAYDREAM WITH INTENT

Now is our time for the luxury of daydreaming. We can wonder at the end of this:

- What do we want to do?
- Where do we want to do?
- Who do we want to do it with?

WHY?

- We've earned it. Simple as that. We can write our dreams down, journal or draw them, allow our mind the time to wander over what it's created and adjust them, turn the colour and the sound up a few notches. And in doing so, not define ourselves by our pre-menopause limits. I revisited my second-phase dreams many times, refining them, adjusting them to fit my new ways of thinking.

- We need to allow the questions we ask of ourselves to draw out what we want for ourselves in our relationship.
- We're removing constraints. If something pops up and takes us by surprise, we have to be accepting not judgemental. This is an opportunity.

CHANGE WITH INTENT

Changes during the menopause mean we become more focused on what we want and are less amenable to those things which impact that. This can be tricky for our partner, as they may be working on pre-menopause time. One of the key indicators we'll give is not simply agreeing to everything they want to do. While this can cause positions to become entrenched, possibly even leading to resentment, for the most part it can be resolved with a simple conversation, possibly two.

WHY?

- Because the menopause takes so long and we've had those tricky symptoms muddying the waters, the changes in us may not have been noticeable to us or our partner. But they may have detected that we're no longer happy to exclusively do what *they* want.

- We'll need to talk about doing what we want taking priority. It can be at a micro, day-to-day level too, affecting the smallest decisions we'll make.
- We need to recognise that this doesn't mean we all swan off and study fine art full-time or island-hop around the Caribbean – some of us might, but we're often working people with lives, responsibilities and constraints. Change needs to be grounded.

TALKING ABOUT SECOND PHASE – YES, WITH INTENT

Now is the time, if it wasn't already evident, for more talking. Haven't we talked enough through the menopause, we may ask? But instead of talking about managing symptoms, changing our social agenda, giving up something and taking something else up instead, this time it's about the fun stuff. What we *want* to do or try.

WHY?

- The next phase of our relationship and the second phase of our womanhood have arrived uncelebrated. There won't be trumpets and bunting, simply a dawning awareness, as our hormones settle into their steady state, that we've made it out of the storm. At this point, therefore, as we change, so must our partner. Only talking can make this possible.
- Within budget or at least comfort level, naturally, we'll be able to think big and work backwards. It's planning – so our

partner will, in all probability, be happy to do the research, connect the dots and draw the project plan.

- As has probably become apparent through this book, Neil and I talk a lot. We've talked about my second phase, too. We still very much talk about what we want to do or achieve in the next five or ten years. It's kept us connected and dreaming of adventures together.

TALKING ABOUT SEX – WITH A LOT OF INTENT

It's the second phase of our intimate life too. Assuming we dealt with our inhibitions after the 'Intimacy' chapter, we're talking about sex. So, it's a time to experiment and take our time to relearn how to please and be pleased by our partner.

WHY?

- We're no longer managing intimacy in the face of our symptoms, we're free of them. We don't have to deal with the anxiety before and hot flushes at the important moments.
- This is a moment of sexual liberation. As mentioned, we're led to believe by popular myth that with the end of the menopause comes the curtain call for our libido. It couldn't be further from the truth, as every woman stepping into their second phase realises. And what a realisation!

GRASP THE POWER – WITH ALL THE INTENT WE HAVE

We're entering a power phase in our life. If we're reading this while in the depths of the maelstrom that is our symptoms, this may seem somewhat fanciful. But our post-menopausal years are our most extraordinary. Our accumulated knowledge and experience, coupled with our renewed focus on our needs and desires, make us formidable. The power is there to be grasped.

WHY?

- Unlike the common belief that women become invisible over a certain age, on the contrary, women become *more* visible. We need to be prepared for the reactions of all those around us to vary in our new-found confidence in who we are. There may be denial in some quarters, as this presents a challenge to the stable, patriarchal way of things, but we know who we are, what we stand for and what our boundaries are – that is, what we're prepared to be pushed on and what we're absolutely not.
- Our partner may need time to adapt, but for men, discovering the new feisty and determined us can be a fascinating pleasure. Likewise, we may also take some time to get used to the new us and the power we wield. We can discover together, free of the menopause.

o o o

The second phase of our womanhood presents us with choices and opportunities that weren't possible before, along with the ability to grasp them. We're shaking off what doesn't serve us and stepping forward into a life of our own making. It's thrilling and exhilarating, and not just a little intoxicating. When it happens, we'll know what to do.

SECOND PHASE: NEIL

LAST TRAIN OUT?

Ask men what happens when the menopause is over, and most won't have a clue. Try it. There's so much focus within available resources, written or practised, on *getting through* the menopause that asking the question about what happens afterwards seems almost pointless. As we've mentioned previously, "well, it all goes back to normal" may be the obvious guess in the scratchy search for an answer. Which, of course, it doesn't. We probably won't even remember what 'normal' once was after so long.

But first, how will it actually end? Bang or whimper? And what's the preferable way in such an instance, anyway? While it's been proven to be better for pain control to pull a plaster off swiftly, we shouldn't diss the appeal of the whimper too quickly. Just as frustrating as knowing when the perimenopause has actually begun, the end is a non-specific affair, too. Just because symptoms have disappeared for a while doesn't mean they won't come back. Like all respectable prog-rock tracks, it fades out and there's a reprise. Or two.

Which means the start of the 'second phase' of a woman's life isn't one of the anniversaries of which we'll be buying a card to acknowledge (unless the menopause was triggered by medical treatment, in which case it probably won't be a cause for celebration at all). Which saves booking a half-decent restaurant too. As we've mentioned, the first phase is puberty to the menopause. There isn't a third phase. So, the second phase could last forty years, give or take, making it longer than the first which is around thirty. That's a heck of a long time for our partner to be engaging in gentle pursuits, as society would have us believe.

Change isn't easy to see when we're two people living together over an unusual eight years or so. We may look back at photos of ourselves before the menopause began and consider how fresh, clear-skinned and energised we seem. But we also look back to the early years of our children's lives, if we have them, and appreciate just how unbearably knackered we look from a relentless commitment to whatever was on TV at 5 a.m., seven days a week.

Just as the menopause will tail off, so the change brought about by it will, to us, slip under the door unnoticed – until a situation arises that reveals it, a test that our partner handles differently; or perhaps it'll be us that they handle differently. At this stage I need to reassure every man reading this that second-phase women are remarkable. We're never going to be forgiven again for thinking it's all about us. Which is quite a favour to be thankful for.

We need to be clear, however, that the second phase of womanhood isn't an imitation of the one male phase. It's not going to herald – in its worst form – an era of irresponsible beer-swilling, foul-mouthed, late-night troublemaking. That's still reserved for those fully grown men who find no embarrassment whatsoever in wearing replica football shirts.

But if in mid-menopause we thought that, as we were changing sheets for the third time in a typically disturbed night, there was nothing to look forward to, we'd be so very wrong.

THANK YOU, GOODNIGHT?

We're assuming here that we're both intent on the relationship having a future. It may be, however, that the dawn of our partner's second phase turns out to be a watershed for her and us. It may come as a surprise, but we're not the only holders of the 'opt out'.

There are several possible scenarios in which our partner may, at this stage, call time:

• Perhaps we haven't been on the journey with them, ignored the menopause, not talked, offered no support, rejected intimacy, kept out of the way. As in, not read this book or acted on any of the suggestions. In which case we've only ourselves to blame.

- It's possible to grow apart during the menopause just as much as it is to grow together. It may only reveal itself when the menopause fades.
- Or it may simply be that the support we've given during the menopause is appreciated, but that what we can offer beyond isn't likely to be. It'll be tough, as we probably considered throughout the menopause that such a situation would never arise.

The menopause doesn't put the need to value our partner and our relationship on hold for the duration. Quite the opposite, in fact, as I hope this book has shown. So, for the last time in these pages, here's what we can do about it.

🎬 NEIL'S ACTION PLAN

MORE MYTHS TO BIN

Yes, we're back to calling out and actively contesting the myths, two of them in this instance. First, the appalling yet ubiquitous myth of female irrelevance after the menopause, the denial of the second phase of womanhood. Second, perpetuated by the first, is the equally dangerous myth of male infallibility in the face of age, our knack of not only defying the years but turning them to our advantage.

WHY?

- They're both not true, not funny and not helpful. Yet they're related, and we'll need to face down both.
- We have a responsibility to do so beyond ourselves – for our family, possibly children, colleagues and friends. We may have a role in enlightening them if they've never had to consider them before.

MORE CHANGES TO MAKE

We'll need to adjust. Kate has described the difference between the first and second phases, caused by the decline in hormones. As men we'll have unconsciously benefitted from this for several decades of our lives. We'll have been looked after. Perhaps not always, perhaps not as much as we'd have liked at times, but it's something we'll notice by its absence. While we might believe *we* perform the chest-thumping kind of looking after, the way will have been paved by our partner to enable us to get on with our careers and attend whatever male-only excursions we're into. It's not going to happen anymore. Our support for our partner doesn't end as the menopause fades – it could be that it's just changing.

WHY?

- It's been a long time coming, and so it's only right that it's time to behave equitably. Arguing that it's an injustice is futile: we've no case.

- We'll be able to understand that what our partner wants isn't necessarily what we expect them to want, or what we want. Which will require openness, honesty and – yes – talking. And as we've covered on many occasions, talking's always good.

MORE PATIENCE TO SHOW

The question for us is, what do we do from here? In the first instance, it's recognising that our partner's menopause is never quite over, rather it's more settled. Our next strategy is, therefore, patience. It means not being frustrated or irritated when some symptoms reappear in the present and suggest they're likely to in the future too.

WHY?

- We've come this far. Really, why would we volunteer to goof it up now?
- The menopause being over doesn't provide an excuse for us to rediscover the less appealing aspects of our character. The moment we utter any form of "oh, for goodness' sake, I thought we were done with all that", we're officially an arse, and quite probably justifying our questionable role in a future together. Because after what may have been eight years of struggle, it's not just unhelpful, it's a display of petulance rightly thought shed a long time ago.

MORE REALITY

Assuming we've been present and involved, we need to understand that we'll both have been changed by the menopause experience. Nothing will go back to the way it was, just as it never has in our lives. It's a time for reappraisal and making plans. Even if they change, or never happen, or we do other things instead. We might leave a notepad and a pen in open view with a list of stuff we'll do, places we'll go, and people we'll avoid in the process.

WHY?

- A post-menopausal mindset will be necessary for us too. We can resolve to unshackle ourselves from attitudes and behaviours that were useful when we were in the metaphorical trenches but have no part to play from here. The siege mentality – whereby everything is against us and we're under attack – must go.
- There are intimacy benefits, being blunt about it. Let's allow ourselves this indulgence in our last bullet point. If our intimacy has suffered, even with our collective will and best efforts, we'll have the perfect opportunity to pursue its reinvigoration. We'll be unburdened by the menstrual cycle and contraception, free to explore and be explored. It's the sort of outcome men would design if they were at the drawing-board stage of sketching out femininity.

o o o

The second phase in a nutshell, therefore, is that it's not what went before; it's something fresh. A newly revealed pleasure for our partner, in so many respects. We've got to hope we can be part of that, in all its manifestations, but it doesn't come as a right. We must earn it. What we forget from our younger years is that in any relationship we always did. Somewhere amid the chaos and unpredictability of the menopause we may have just lost sight of that, but it's time we rediscovered what a fantastic relationship needs when it's not under siege, when the road is open. Which from here, for us together, it very much is.

CLOSE

As the authors, here are our closing thoughts.

We all love things in our lives to be easy and simple. Yet the menopause isn't *just* an end, as is so often portrayed, with nothing beyond. Nor is it *just* a beginning, leading nowhere in particular. It's an end, a transition *and* a beginning. Each stage has its features and its characteristics, all equally worthy of understanding. Only by seeing it as a whole, connected to the rest of our lives, can we really begin to understand and manage it.

We've interwoven our thoughts on a range of matters related to the menopause because we've spent three quarters of our sixteen years together with it in our relationship; lurking at first, then raging, and then slithering away again. We've not been able to bookmark the beginning and end, but it feels now as we write this book that it's been ever-present. Either because the early part of our time together involved the birth and early years of our two daughters, especially challenging for two people who had known fairly limited responsibility (and not a few lost weekends) to this point, or because shortly thereafter we were expecting the arrival of the menopause. Like a not-so-welcome guest we'd invited but forgotten to say when. On tenterhooks.

From the way we've told the story, you may be forgiven for thinking it was, for us, a breeze. It wasn't. We hope it's spoken to you as adults trying to simply make sense of it all. While there's been an attempt at flow in the way the chapters have been arranged, as we've suggested it's somewhat circular. The book ends when the menopause ends, but we almost felt as though we needed to present each chapter at the same time.

But the lightness you may detect is, perhaps, misleading. It stems from our early advice in this book, to *talk and keep talking*. We've never held back together, nor been apprehensive about addressing anything difficult. Probably because we'd been burned in the past by avoiding saying what needed to be said. Or, perhaps, being a little older, a little wiser (we hope), and not having time any longer for the darkness and claustrophobia of rabbit holes. But that said, the menopause has been a learning experience throughout, and continues to be.

As we've identified, being in a close relationship means we're both experiencing the menopause. Which means committing to handling it together is a superpower. Just as we did, you'll both get things wrong, make poor decisions, regret taking a few paths you wish you'd checked beforehand, and just at times be plain unlucky. We're human beings and therefore fundamentally vulnerable. And the menopause brings out the most vulnerable in us all, female and male.

If you're a woman approaching or at menopausal age and are reading this and you're in a stable relationship, your partner needs to read it too. It's not just for you to do the research and provide the 'management summary' for when he's got the time or patience. Because the patience needed for this must be shared.

If you're the man in this relationship reading it, well done; if you're reading it *before* your partner, full respect. For women there's probably too much information and guidance available in the market, for men nowhere near enough. As we explored, reliance on mainstream media to inform is a questionable tactic, to be avoided if possible. We can only hope they'll get it right eventually. The pharmaceutical lobby is influential in this space, too. They have products to sell, after all. But for couples? There's almost no guidance at all. Which is why we decided to write this book. That was a choice we made together too.

We want to thank you for reading this book. Ultimately, we hope you take something from it that helps or works for you, individually and together, and the process brings you closer.

For you both, and for the wider world in which the menopause continues its struggle to be taken seriously, we rather hope we've started something.

As for continuing it, that's now up to you.

NOTES AND REFERENCES

The following contains references to data and statements made in the book, with suggestions for further reading. We've tried to capture everything in which you may be interested but can't claim it to be exhaustive.

The menopause is still very much a 'live' issue with new research and perspectives regularly being published.

In terms of journals, *Post Reproductive Health*, the journal of the British Menopause Society, published by Sage (www.journals.sagepub.com/home/min), is often interesting. You need to be a member of the Society to receive it.

INTRODUCTION

A description of the andropause – what it is, what it's not and how it's treated – can be found at:
"The 'Male Menopause'", *NHS UK*: https://www.nhs.uk/conditions/male-menopause/.

WHAT IS THE MENOPAUSE?

An easy read, written by a highly respected clinician, who is also the former Chair of the British Menopause Society:

Kathy Abernethy, *Menopause the one-stop guide: A practical guide to understanding and dealing with the menopause* (London: Profile Books, 2018).

This bestselling book, written in a human and approachable style, covers all aspects of menopause and its treatment:
Dr Jen Gunter, *The Menopause Manifesto* (London: Piatkus, 2021).

Another excellent and detailed 'everything you need to know' guide is:
Pat Wingert and Barbara Kantrowitz, *The Menopause Book* (New York: Workman Publishing Company, 2018).

For a more natural explanation of what's going on – written by the leading light on menopause awareness (2021 edition, first published 2001):
Christiane Northrup, M.D., *The Wisdom of Menopause, Creating Physical and Emotional Health During the Change* (London: Hay House, 2021).

A useful and accessible summary for men and women alike – albeit one titled for men – is contained in:
Ruth Devlin, *Men.... Let's Talk Menopause* (London: Practical Inspiration Publishing, 2019).

75 per cent of women have hot flushes (flashes) – but if you

are waiting for one before you get a diagnosis, they may never occur, as this article explains:

"Menopause FAQs: Hot flashes", *North American Menopause Society*, 2023:

https://www.menopause.org/for-women/
menopause-faqs-hot-flashes

PERCEPTIONS

For detailed and insightful studies of the history of menopause and the perception of women through the ages, both of the following are comprehensive and well researched. Mattern's book is more academic:

Louise Foxcroft, *Hot Flushes, Cold Science: A History of the Modern Menopause* (London: Granta, 2009).

Susan P. Mattern, *The Slow Moon Climbs: The Science, History and Meaning of Menopause* (Princeton, New Jersey: Princeton University Press, 2019).

For an incredible walk through the history of medicine's bias against women and the resulting issues we see and perceptions we have about female health and our ability to be medical practitioners:

Elinor Cleghorn, *Unwell Women: A Journey Through Medicine and Myth in a Man-Made World* (UK. Orion, 2021).

A useful summary of female economic power can be found in the following – there are a variety of other accessible articles: Bridget Brennan, "What Every Marketer Should Know About Women's Economic Power", *Forbes*, 20 Oct 2022: https://www.forbes.com/sites/bridgetbrennan/2022/10/20/what-every-marketer-should-know-about-womens-economic-power/?sh=1059ea294d4c.

This is Kate's all-time favourite book about what women's contribution to the world economy is and could be:
Linda Scott, *The Double X Economy, The epic potential of empowering women* (London: Faber & Faber, 2020).

The age-old male preference for 'younger women' is evidenced in a study from 2020 – but interestingly it notes this has become less marked with progress in gender equality: Kathryn Walter, Daniel Conroy-Beam and Maja Zupančič, "Sex Differences in Mate Preferences Across 45 Countries: A Large-Scale Replication", *Psychological Science*, Vol 31 Issue 4, 20 March 2020.

Meanwhile, the average age gap between heterosexual couples according to a study spanning seventy years of data is two to four years, as found in:
Martin Kolk, *Age Differences in Unions: Continuity and Divergence in Sweden between 1932 and 2007* (Stockholm: Stockholm Research Reports in Demography, 2013).

For an eye-opening explanation of male dominance and lack of female awareness in advertising and the resulting manipulation and 'brandsplaining':
Jane Cunningham & Philippa Roberts, *Brandsplaining: Why marketing is still sexist & how to fix it* (London: Penguin Business 2021).

If you like the above book, there is also:
Jane Cunningham & Philippa Roberts, *Inside her pretty little head* (London: Marshall Cavendish Business, 2012).

TALKING

The *Future Men Survey* conducted by YouGov in 2018 on behalf of the UK charity Working with Men was revealing in terms of how men feel about themselves, and expectations upon them to 'man up' when faced with emotional challenges: https://futuremen.org/future-men-2018-survey/

This is an interesting article that looks at issues related to men's unwillingness to talk about their emotions:
Sean McAllister, "Why don't men talk about their feelings?" *Zurich*, 6 Oct 2022: https://www.zurich.com/en/media/magazine/2021/tackling-the-silence-why-dont-men-talk-about-their-feelings

There's a huge amount written about toxic masculinity in

which the myth of the 'strong, silent type' is explored (and dismantled) – an example worth exploring is:
Jared Yates Sexton, *The Man They Wanted Me to Be: Toxic masculinity and a crisis of our own making* (Berkeley: Counterpoint, 2019).

'Mansplaining' as a term originated in this essay – it's here with a new intro:
Rebecca Solnit, "Men Explain Things to Me", *Guernica*, 20 August 2012: https://www.guernicamag.com/rebecca-solnit-men-explain-things-to-me/

'Mansplaining' can best be described in a single chart that went viral on social media in 2018, and is discussed here:
Kim Goodwin, "Mansplaining explained in one simple chart", *BBC*, 29 July 2018:
https://www.bbc.com/worklife/article/20180727-mansplaining-explained-in-one-chart

This article focusses on men's need to explain things to women:
Kate Manne, "Why are men still explaining things to women?" *New York Times*, 9 Sept 2020:
https://www.nytimes.com/2020/09/09/us/why-are-men-still-explaining-things-to-women-mansplaining-authority-gender.html

In respect of our tendency to complete a half-told story, to fill in the gaps, this can be explained by the 'illusion of explanatory depth' (IOED), which describes our belief that we understand more about the world than we actually do. Here's a brief introduction:
https://www.edge.org/response-detail/27117

For an analysis of brilliance as a male trait, see this article: "Men More Likely Than Women to Be Seen as Brilliant", *New York University*, 20 October 2020:
https://www.nyu.edu/about/news-publications/news/2020/july/men-more-likely-than-women-to-be-seen-as-brilliant-.html

For a practical guide to listening, this piece is useful:
Adam Bryant, "How to be a better listener", *New York Times*, undated:
https://www.nytimes.com/guides/smarterliving/be-a-better-listener

We did say there wasn't a downside to being a good listener, but there are several articles suggesting there is. Here's a good example:
Sophie Dembling, "Why I Worry About Being a Good Listener", *Psychology Today*, 15 June 2016: https://www.psychologytoday.com/gb/blog/the-introverts-corner/201606/why-i-worry-about-being-good-listener

When looking at the potential impact of lack of communication on relationship breakdown, this article from *Cosmopolitan* (OK, it's not an academic article) is interesting as not only is poor communication mentioned, but nine out of the ten reasons given could be attributed to the menopause:
Laura Beck, "10 Super-Common Reasons Couples in Long-Term Relationships Break Up", *Cosmopolitan*, 8 May 2016 https://www.cosmopolitan.com/sex-love/news/a58127/reasons-long-term-couples-break-up/.

EXPECTATIONS

It's been proven that babies show surprise and dismay before they can even talk:
University of Missouri-Columbia, "Babies are born with 'intuitive physics' knowledge, says researcher", *Science Daily*, 25 Jan 2012: https://www.sciencedaily.com/releases/2012/01/120124113051.htm

A recent book about women's expectations of 'having it all':
Emma Gannon, *The Success Myth: Our obsession with achievement is a trap. This is how to break free* (London: Torva, 2023).

For an understanding of what's going on in your brain during the menopause:

Dr Louann Brizedine, *The Upgrade: How the female brain gets stronger and better in midlife and beyond* (London: Hay House, 2022).

For a discussion of humans as pattern-seeking creatures, see: Michael Shermer, "We Are the World", *Los Angeles Times*, 6 Feb 2000:
https://www.latimes.com/archives/la-xpm-2000-feb-06-bk-61427-story.html

For the difference between anxiety and depression see: Pablo Vandenebeele, "What's the difference between anxiety and depression?" *BUPA*, 31 Mar 2021: https://www.bupa.co.uk/newsroom/ourviews/anxiety-depression

The highest rates of suicide amongst women in the UK is between the ages of 45–49 closely followed by ages 50–54: "Suicide Statistics", *House of Commons Library*, Dec 2022: https://commonslibrary.parliament.uk/research-briefings/cbp-7749/

The perceptions around women and pain are discussed in *Unwell Women*, referenced above. This article is also interesting:
Edmund Keogh, "Do men have a higher pain threshold than men, or are they just a bit emotionally repressed?" *The Conversation*, May 2014:

https://theconversation.com/do-men-have-a-higher-
threshold-for-pain-or-are-they-just-a-bit-emotionally-
repressed-25681

The impact of perceived stereotypes in medicine, and the
need for women to prove their level of illness in comparison
to men to receive comparable treatment, is discussed in this
excellent podcast:
Ivan Beckley, Emma Barnaby, Yero Timi-Biu, Anishka Sharma
and Tej Adeleye: "The Bias Diagnosis, Gender injustice in
healthcare", *Audible*, 2021.

This article also explains why women in acute or chronic
pain are often underdiagnosed and undertreated:
Fortesa Latifi, "The Pain Gap: Why Women's Pain is
Undertreated", *Healthy Women*, 26 July 2021: https://
www.healthywomen.org/condition/pain-gap-womens-pain-
undertreated

LIFESTYLE

There are numerous studies about increased weight gain
during menopause, many contradicting each other. This
infographic from *Women's Health Concern*, the patient arm
of the *British Menopause Society*, highlights the impact of
obesity on breast cancer risk and the benefit of exercising:

"Understanding the risks of breast cancer", *Women's Health Concern*, Nov 2015:
https://www.womens-health-concern.org/wp-content/uploads/2019/10/WHC-UnderstandingRisksofBreastCancer-MARCH2017.pdf

Kate talks about eating low-sugar fruits – there's more here: Jordan Davidson, "The 10 Healthiest Low-Sugar Fruits You Should Be Eating", *Good Housekeeping*, 14 Oct 2020:
https://www.goodhousekeeping.com/health/diet-nutrition/a20705822/healthiest-low-sugar-fruits/

For information around osteoporosis during and after the menopause, this paper from *Women's Health Concern* is useful:
"Osteoporosis – bone health after menopause", *Women's Health Concern*, 2021:
https://www.womens-health-concern.org/wp-content/uploads/2022/12/19-WHC-FACTSHEET-Osteoporosis-Bone-NOV2022-B.pdf

Alternatively, the Endocrine Society website gives a simple explanation:
"Menopause and Bone Loss", *Endocrine Society,* 24 Jan 2022:
https://www.endocrine.org/patient-engagement/endocrine-library/menopause-and-bone-loss

If you would like information on why women are at greater risk of heart disease during and after the menopause, this is an excellent simple explanation:

"Menopause and Heart Disease", *British Heart Foundation*: https://www.bhf.org.uk/informationsup-port/support/women-with-a-heart-condition/menopause-and-heart-disease

If you would like information on why focusing on keeping fit and healthy is important during the menopause and how diabetes can be avoided, this will help:

"Menopause and Diabetes", *Diabetes UK* https://www.dia-betes.org.uk/guide-to-diabetes/life-with-diabetes/menopause

An accessible read with super tips on staying fit and healthy during the menopause (and at any other time too) can be found in:

Stacey T. Sims, *Next Level: Your Guide to Kicking Ass, Feeling Great, and Crushing Goals Through Menopause and Beyond* (New York: Rodale Books, 2021).

MOODS

Kate talks about splashing very cold water on your face to calm down and take control in moments of anxiety. It's part of the TIPP group of techniques – temperature, intense exercise, paced breathing and progressive muscle relaxation.

A good explanation can be found here:

"The TIPP technique", *Norfolk and Suffolk NHS Foundation Trust*: https://www.youtube.com/watch?v=8nVady7A3Qo

NIGHT AND DAY

Sleep deprivation appears to have been first documented as an effective torture by Italian lawyer Hippolytus de Marsiliis (1451–1529), thereby ensuring it was added to the tools of the Inquisition. It was also used during the witch trials in Europe (1500–1660) to get women to admit to witchcraft. Here's a useful summary:

Jeff Mann, "A brief history of sleep deprivation and torture", *Sleep Junkies*, 9 Dec 2022: https://sleepjunkies.com/sleep-deprivation-and-torture-a-brief-history/

The term we used "fog of menopause" is based on the term "fog of war", first used by the Prussian military analyst Carl von Clausewitz in his book *Vom Kriege* (posthumously published in 1837).

We're not psychologists and so getting into the science of whether women and men think differently is a rabbit hole we'll avoid on this occasion, despite having made the odd quip about men having a more binary approach. However, this article is worth a read, as it references that men tend to focus on one task:

Rebecca Shambaugh, "Different Brains, Different Behaviors: Why Women Lead Differently Than Men", *Huffpost*, 17 March 2016: https://www.huffpost.com/entry/different-brains-differen_b_9480952.

It's easy to assume that maternity and parental leave has been in existence for many years. Yet it wasn't until 1993 in the UK that all women qualified. Men were only entitled to paid paternity leave from 2003. More information can be found here:

"Maternity (and Paternity) Leave and Pay", *Striking Women*: https://www.striking-women.org/module/workplace-issues-past-and-present/maternity-and-paternity-leave-and-pay

And here too:

Alice Azania-Jarvis, "The Timeline: Maternity Leave", *The Independent*, 22 Oct 2010: https://www.independent.co.uk/life-style/health-and-families/features/the-timeline-maternity-leave-2113236.html

A 'bestselling' take on sleep can be found in:

Matthew Walker, *Why We Sleep: The New Science of Sleep and Dreams* (London: Penguin, 2018).

INTIMACY

Kate references the importance of gestures between us – this book talks about showing connection in five specific ways depending on your preference:
Gary Chapman, *The 5 Love Languages, The Secret to Love That Lasts* (Chicago: Northfield Publishing, 2010).

The following recent book about sex emphasises the importance of talking about it:
Dr Emily Morse, *Smart Sex: How to Boost Your Sex IQ and Own Your Pleasure* (London: HQ, 2023).

This is an excellent book about intimacy for the menopause and all other time:
Dr Karen Gurney, *Mind the Gap: The truth about desire and how to futureproof your sex life* (London: Headline Publishing Group, 2020).

Vaginal dryness can be excruciatingly painful. If this is your experience, the following is highly recommend reading:
Jane Lewis, *Me & My Menopausal Vagina, Living with vaginal atrophy* (UK: PAL Books, 2018).

Professor Jennifer Chatman University of California-Berkeley conducted research in 2017 into whether there was a point at which flattery becomes ineffective through being overdone. It showed that there's no such point – flattery never fails to stop working.

SECOND PHASE

Christiane Northrup's book (mentioned earlier) references the reasons why before the menopause women prioritise the safety and wellbeing of others over themselves.

Pulling off a plaster quickly has been proven to be better than removing it slowly – here's a good example of such a study: Jeremy S Furyk, Carl J O'Kane, Peter J Aitken, Colin J Banks and David A Kault, "Fast versus slow bandaid removal: a randomised trial", *Medical Journal of Australia*, 191 (11), 7 December 2009: https://www.mja.com.au/journal/2009/191/11/fast-versus-slow-bandaid-removal-randomised-trial

Of course, we couldn't let this section pass without mentioning Kate's book, which is very much focussed on the second phase:
Kate Usher, *Your Second Phase: Reclaiming work and relationships during and after menopause* (London: LID Business Publishing, 2020).

CLOSE

There are plenty of resources with an analysis of the value of the global HRT market – here's an example:

"Global Hormone Replacement Theary (HRT) Market", *Fortune Business Insights*, Feb 2022: https://www.fortunebusinessinsights.com/hormone-replacement-therapy-hrt-market-102543

ABOUT THE AUTHORS

At the time of writing this book, Neil and Kate have been married for sixteen years and live with their teenage daughters and their dog in London, UK.

Kate is a menopause coach and gender equity consultant, working for over ten years with women and organisations to create modern menopause conversations that enable women to stay in their chosen careers and achieve their professional ambitions. Prior to this she has twenty years' experience leading IT transformation projects in FTSE100 organisations. Kate's first book *Your Second Phase: Reclaiming work and relationships during and after menopause* was shortlisted for the Business Book of the Year award in 2020.

Neil is a property, workplace and change leader with over thirty years' experience, working within and advising multinational clients on all aspects of finding, securing, creating and managing fantastic places to work. He's been writing, blogging and talking about work and the workplace for more than a decade, and has published four books to date. His work mixes organisational and business thinking with music, literature and philosophy, and always brings a much-needed cutting edge. He's been known to do performance poetry too.

ALSO BY KATE USHER

Your Second Phase: Reclaiming work and relationships during and after menopause (London: LID Publishing, 2020)

ALSO BY NEIL USHER

The Elemental Workplace (London: LID Publishing, 2018)
Elemental Change (London: LID Publishing, 2020)
Unf*cking Work (Winchester: Zero Books, 2022)
Workspace Made Easy with Kursty Groves (London: Routledge, 2024)

ACKNOWLEDGEMENTS

Thanks to Sugandi Aravinth, Ella Aziz, Sheryl Andrews, Tracey Baum, Katherine Bellchambers, Helen Blunden, Sue Brooks, Jennifer Bryan, Hannah Edwards, Carol Elam, Susan Furber, Giverney Harman, Pauline Hill, Gill McKay, Fiona Scott, Taz Thornton and Fiona Tribe for help, encouragement and advice in helping bring this book to life.

THE BACK PAGES

If you've enjoyed this book and perhaps found it useful – or maybe haven't – and wish to get in touch, please feel free to do so:

KATE

Web:	www.menopauseinbusiness.com
X:	@menoinbusiness
LinkedIn:	linkedin.com/in/kateusher/
Instagram:	instagram.com/kateushermenopause/
Email:	kate@menopauseinbusiness.com

NEIL

X:	@workessence
LinkedIn:	linkedin.com/in/neilusher/
Instagram:	instagram.com/workessence/
Email:	neilusher@hotmail.com

Reviews and comment on social media – good, bad or ugly – are always massively appreciated.

If you wish to cite this book (and thank you if you do!):

Kate Usher and Neil Usher, *A Couple's Guide to Menopause: Navigating the Change Together* (London: Hero, 2024).

Look out for the second volume where we'll be considering how to manage the menopause from a woman's and a man's perspective in the workplace. Coming soon.